HOW TO FEEL LESS ANXIOUS

CHRISTINA NEAL

vie

HOW TO FEEL LESS ANXIOUS

Design by Luci Ward

An Hachette UK Company
www.hachette.co.uk

Summersdale Publishers Ltd
Part of Octopus Publishing Group Limited
Carmelite House
50 Victoria Embankment
LONDON
EC4Y 0DZ

www.summersdale.com

Printed and bound in China

ISBN: 978-1-78783-545-0

DISCLAIMER
The author and the publisher cannot accept responsibility for any misuse or misunderstanding of any information contained herein, or any loss, damage or injury, be it health, financial or otherwise, suffered by any individual or group acting upon or relying on information contained herein. None of the views or suggestions in this book is intended to replace medical opinion from a doctor who is familiar with your particular circumstances. If you have concerns about your health, please seek professional advice.

Contents

Introduction

It's natural for all of us to worry from time to time. Usually, our anxious thoughts will pass, or the everyday things that have caused concern will work themselves out in the end. However, constant worrying or feeling fearful for much of the time could be a sign of anxiety. It's important to address anxiety and worry, as they can have a detrimental effect on our health in the long term. It can help to know you're not alone. The World Health Organization (WHO) reports that one in 13 people globally suffers from anxiety. The Anxiety and Depression Association of America claims that anxiety disorder is the most common mental illness in the United States, with approximately 40 million Americans experiencing the condition. In the UK, the charity Anxiety UK says that approximately three million people are suffering from an anxiety disorder.

While it can seem very real and frightening at the time, it's reassuring to know that worry and anxiety can be controlled and managed. Understanding what anxiety is and practising different techniques to cope with your anxiety and worry are the first steps toward calming your mind. This book will explore anxiety and worry to give you a better understanding of what might be triggering your anxious thoughts, reveal how you can manage your mindset and ultimately, help you to relieve anxious feelings.
The following pages are packed with tips and tricks to calm yourself, help you to breathe and think more clearly and take life in your stride, rather than feeling that constant buzz of an overly busy brain.
So, take a step back from your fears, take a few deep breaths and read on with an open mind...

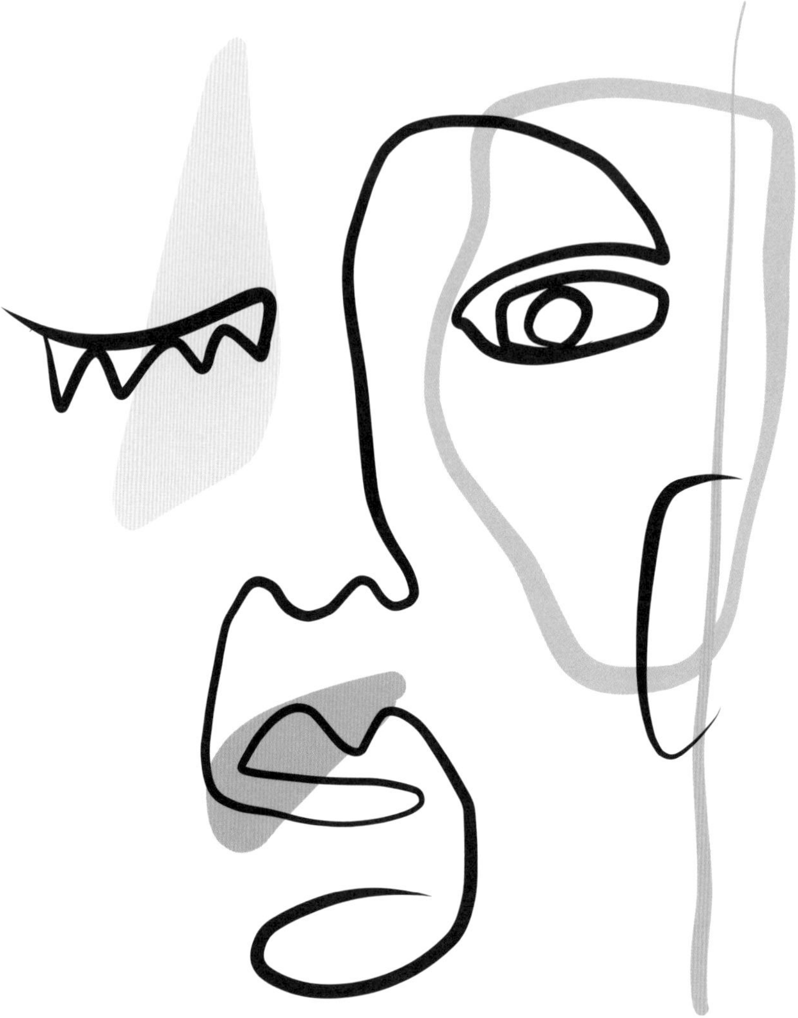

PART ONE:
UNDERSTANDING ANXIETY

So, what is anxiety? Anxiety is a feeling of fear, unease or worry that can be mild or severe. A person who is suffering from anxiety may find that their worries grow out of proportion to a problem or situation, and feelings can become extremely intense. A sense of feeling overwhelmed can prevail and the person may no longer be able to think clearly. Their thoughts may be irrational and even unfounded, but they can seem very genuine at the time. There are various types of anxiety. According to criteria outlined in *The Diagnostic and Statistical Manual of Mental Disorders*, Fifth Edition, professionals look for excessive worry combined with physical symptoms, such as impaired concentration, irritability and difficulty sleeping, to name just a few. Anxiety can manifest in many different ways, and not everyone finds it helpful to put a label on their own experience, but it can be useful to understand the most common kinds to see if you identify with one type over another.

Some of the more common kinds of anxiety are:

- **General Anxiety Disorder (GAD)** – having regular concerns about many everyday aspects of your life.
- **Social Anxiety Disorder** – a fear of social situations such as parties or any gathering where you have to talk to and interact with others.
- **Panic Disorder** – a symptom of panic disorder is a panic attack. Panic attacks are an exaggeration of your body's natural response to stress or danger. Symptoms include a pounding heart, feeling faint, dizzy, sick and very hot or cold.
- **Phobias** – an extreme fear of an object or situation.
- Other types include health anxiety or hypochondria (an obsession about the possibility of being ill), body dysmorphic disorder (an obsession with your appearance and trying to be physically perfect) and Perinatal Anxiety, which can occur during pregnancy or after having a baby.

In this chapter, we look at various triggers for anxiety and begin to look at strategies to deal with them. Part of the solution to managing anxiety is simply to recognize and understand signs and symptoms, so that you are better placed to cope with anxious feelings when they arise.

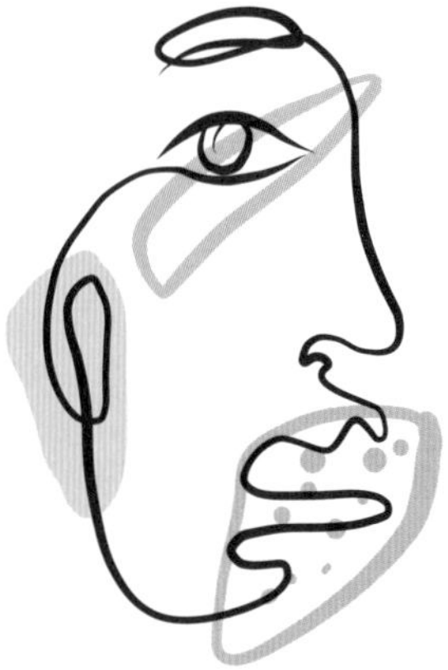

Thoughts are just thoughts

Remember that negative thoughts are just that – thoughts – and not necessarily based on reality or what might happen. Next time a negative thought creeps in, write it down, read it back to yourself and question whether or not it's really true. Writing these thoughts down will enable you to think about them in a more rational way and you may then find you have an entirely different perspective.

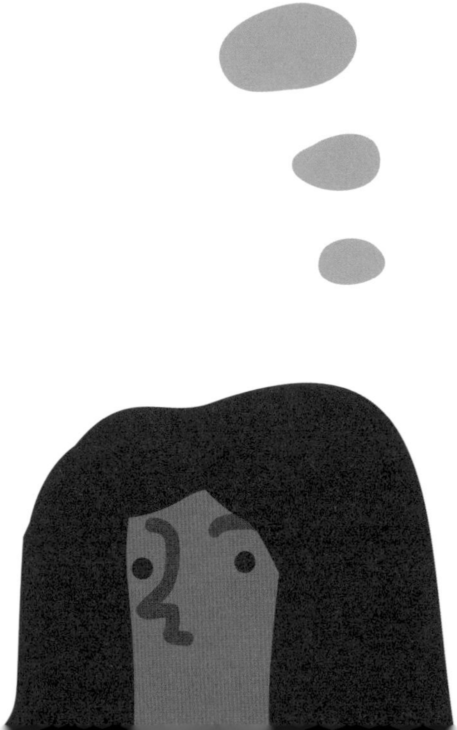

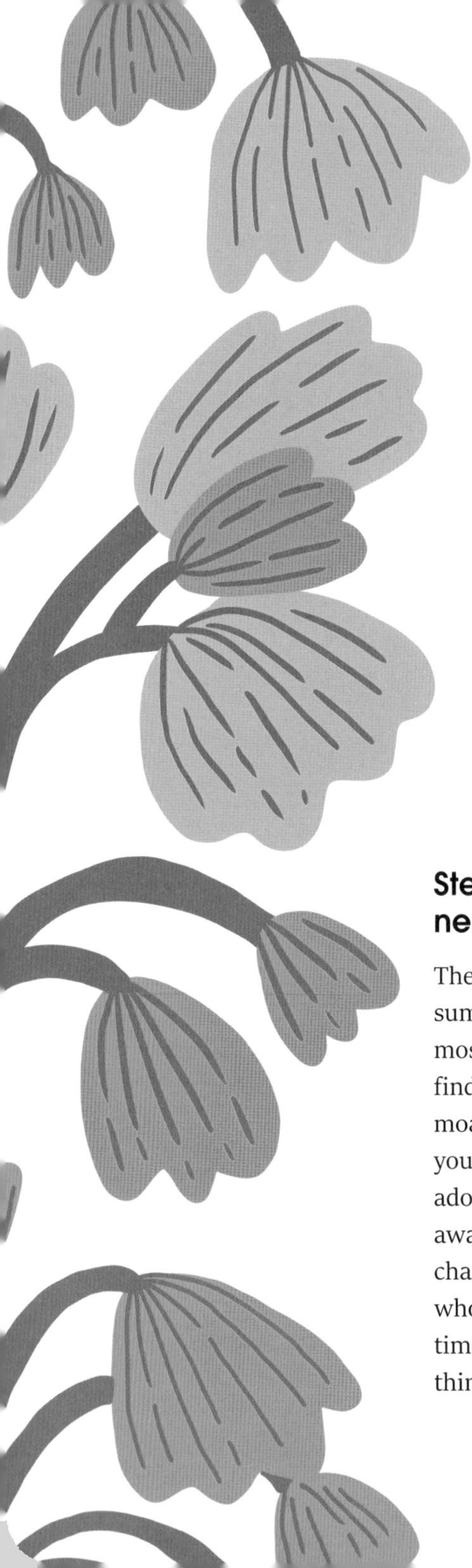

Steer clear of negative people

There is an expression: "You are the sum of the five people you spend the most time with." This is so true. If you find yourself surrounded by negative, moaning and unhappy individuals, you will, in time, start to find yourself adopting their negative behaviour. Be aware of how your thoughts start to change when you are around others who have a negative attitude. The more time you spend worrying or dreading things, the more you'll be held back.

Try to eliminate negative people from your life. Anyone who constantly moans but doesn't do anything to make their own life better, or anyone who tells you that something can't be done or you're wasting your time, is not going to help you improve your own mindset. Try to surround yourself with upbeat, positive "can-do" people and you will find that their energy and enthusiasm will have an uplifting effect on you.

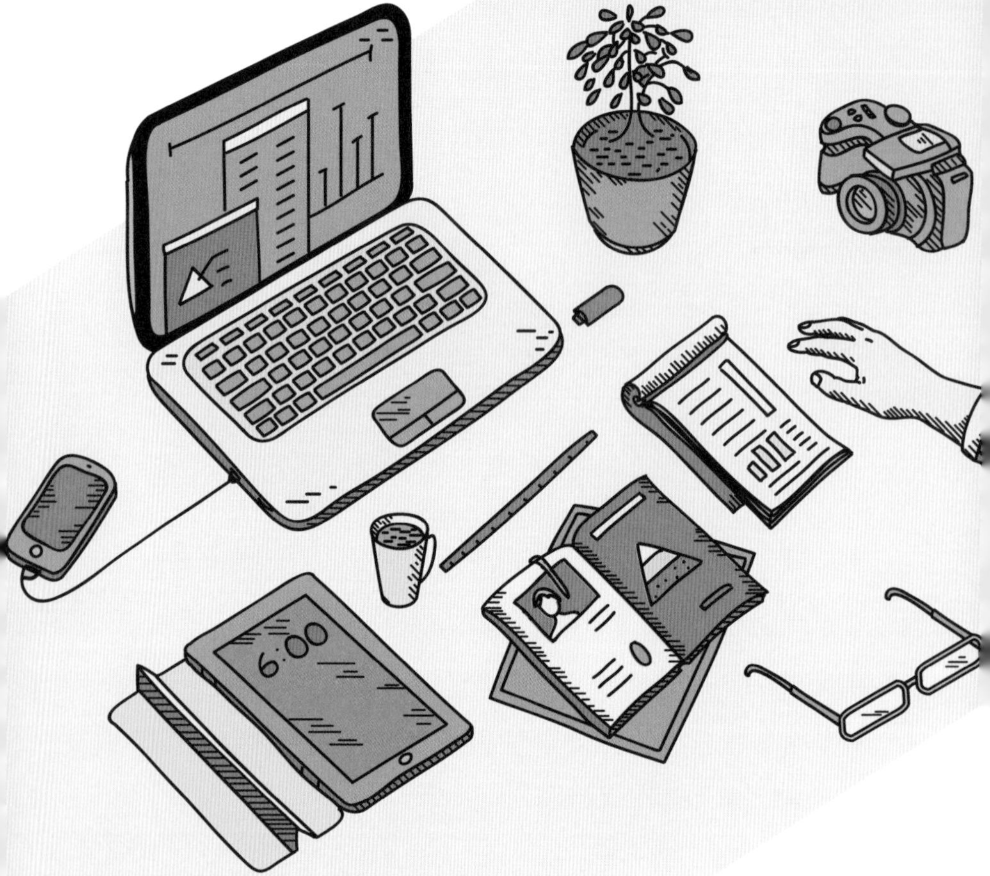

Track your triggers

In order to understand what is causing your anxiety, it may be worth keeping a diary of your daily activities and how you are feeling. This will help you to identify which activities or tasks are triggering negative thoughts and behaviours; once you know what these are, you might be able to eradicate some of them.

OUR ANXIETY DOES NOT COME FROM THINKING ABOUT THE FUTURE, BUT FROM WANTING TO CONTROL IT

Do not anticipate trouble or worry about what may never happen. Keep in the sunlight.

Benjamin Franklin

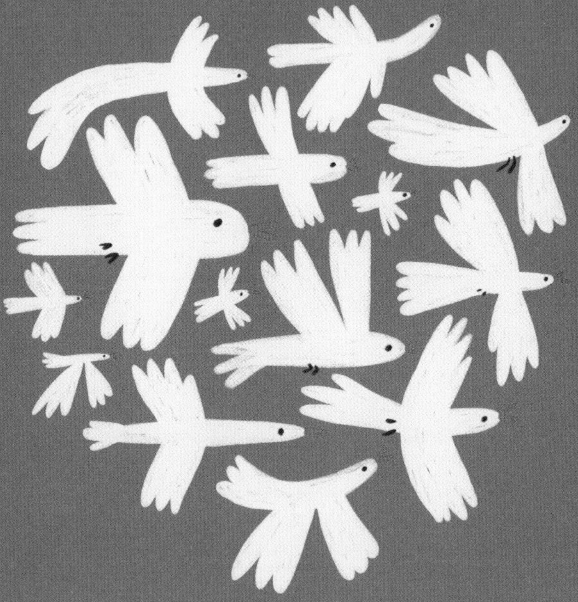

We can't know our future

If you worry about where you'll be or what might happen in a few years' time, your thoughts are more likely to spiral out of control as you weigh up what could go wrong or worry about not achieving your goals. Restore calm by taking a few deep breaths and focusing on what you are doing now. Live in the moment – take in everything that surrounds you: the sights, sounds and smells and the world going about its business.

Accept how you're feeling

Next time you feel anxiety or even panic setting in, don't try to convince yourself it's not happening, or it shouldn't happen. Allow the feelings to wash over you. Don't beat yourself up about the fact that you're feeling this way – you don't have to be perfect. Acknowledge that it is happening and don't tell yourself you should get over it. You can try to repeat affirmations that may make you feel better or remind yourself of other occasions when you managed to get through feeling like this. Repeat positive statements until you start to feel the anxiety subsiding. Take care of yourself afterward, too. You may want to have a drink of water, rest for a while or talk to someone. Be kind to yourself.

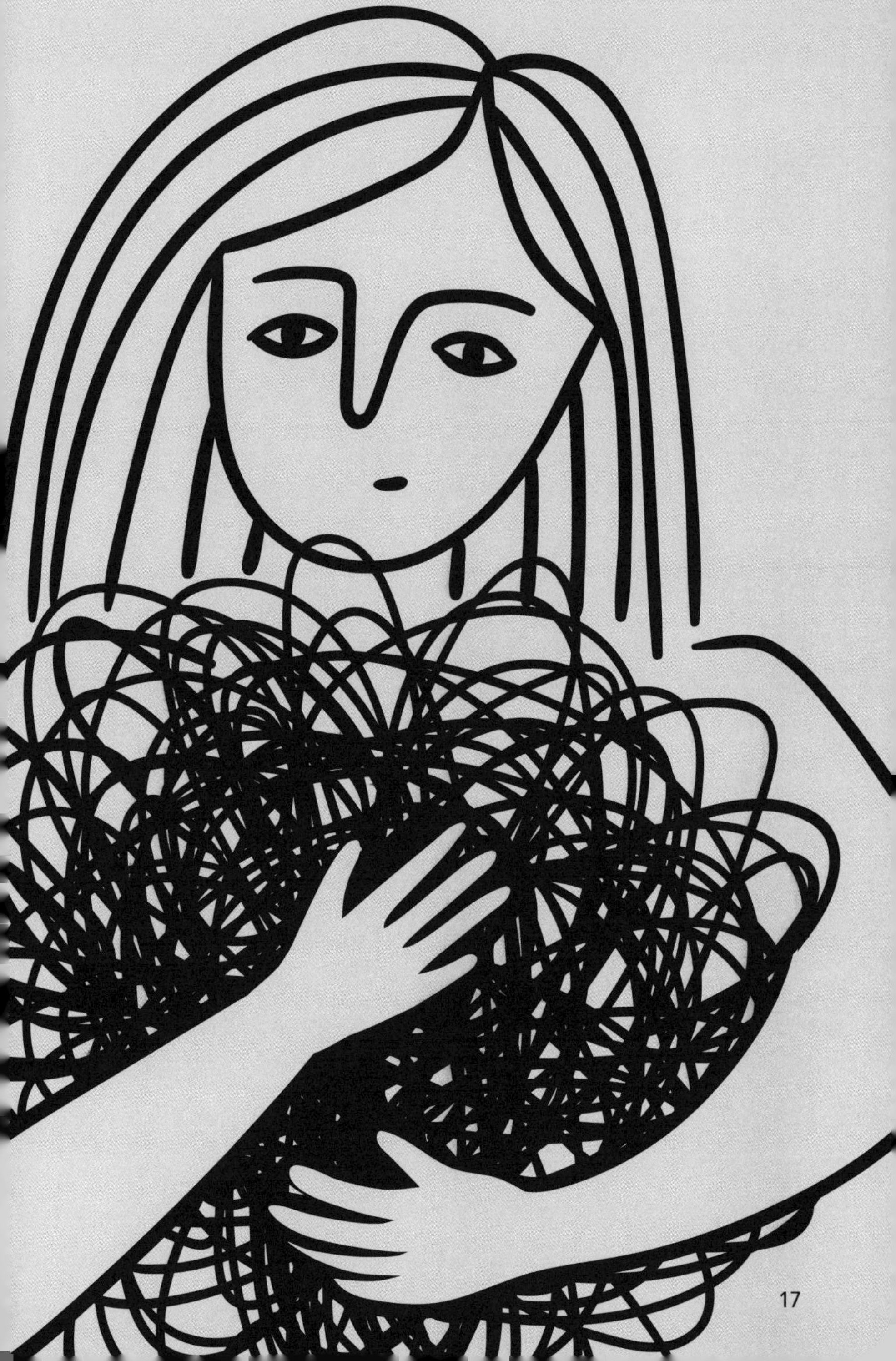

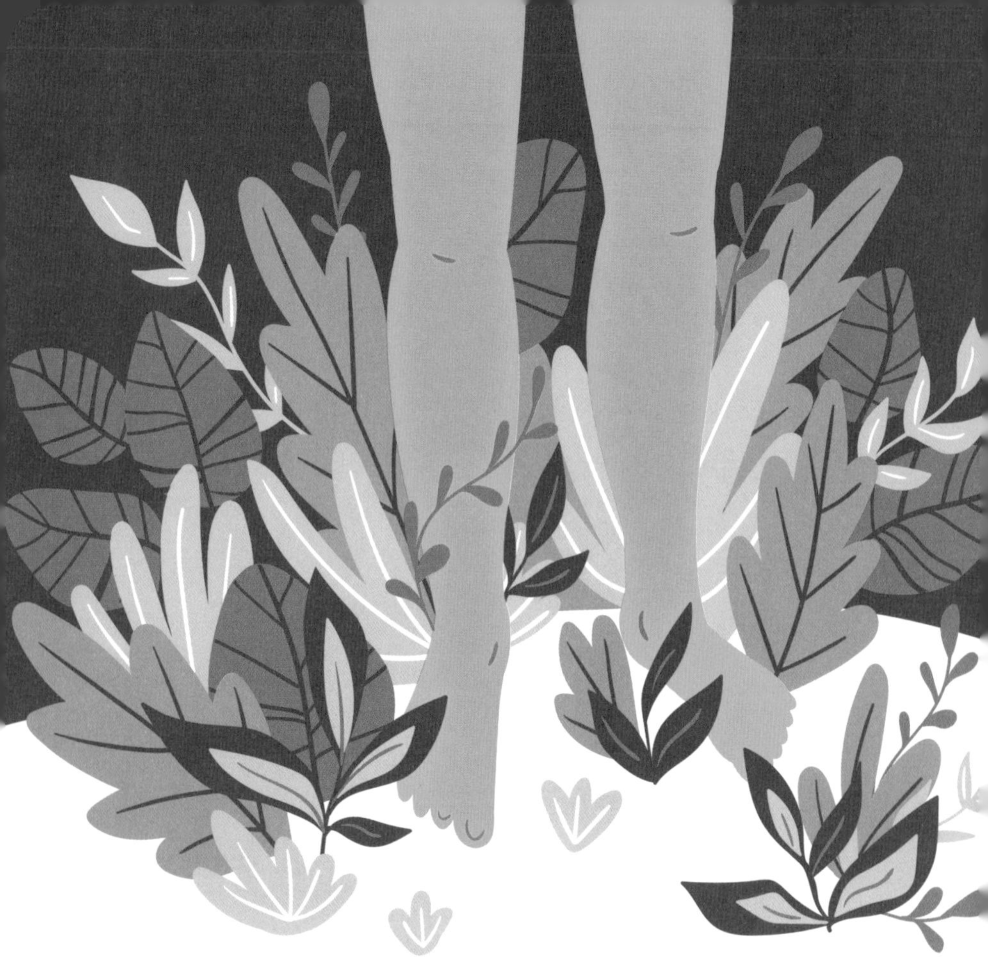

Celebrate where you are and be thankful for where you are going

Look for the positive

Negative thoughts can spin out of control if you're not careful. One adverse thought can lead to another and before you know it, you've built yourself into a distressed state where you may be starting to panic. Curb this type of thinking by countering a negative thought with a positive one. If you make a mistake for instance, rather than feeling bad about it, tell yourself that you've learned something from the mistake. If something goes wrong, look for a solution rather than focusing on what went wrong.

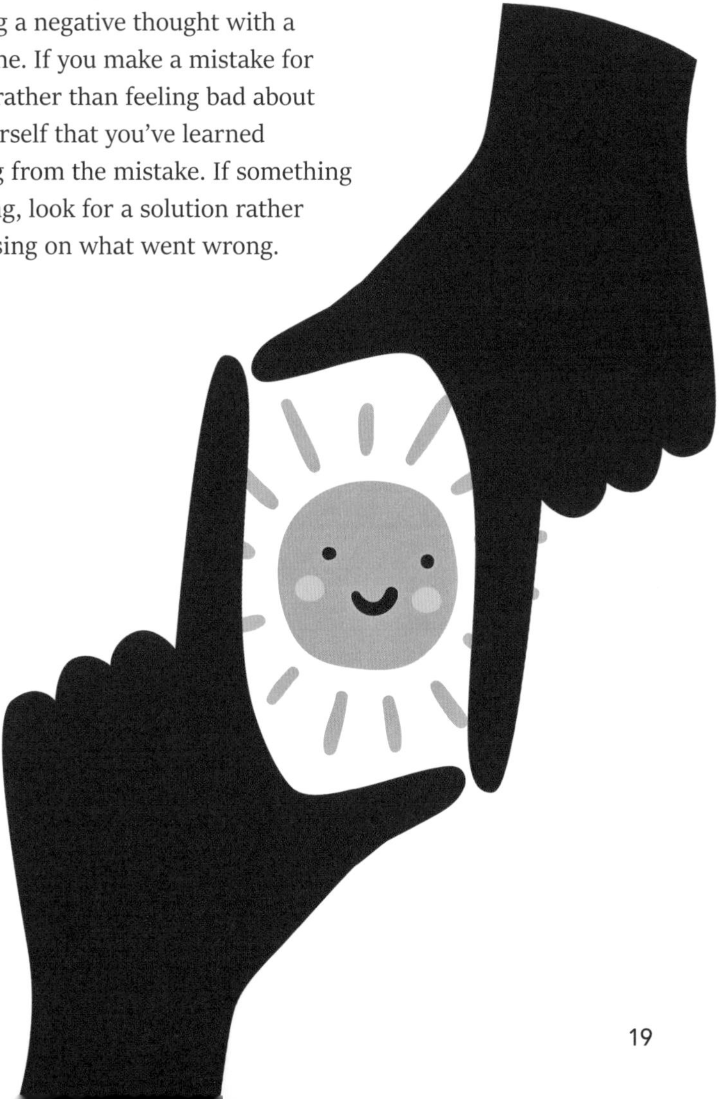

YOU HAVE TWO CHOICES: TO CONTROL YOUR MIND OR TO LET YOUR MIND CONTROL YOU.

Paulo Coelho

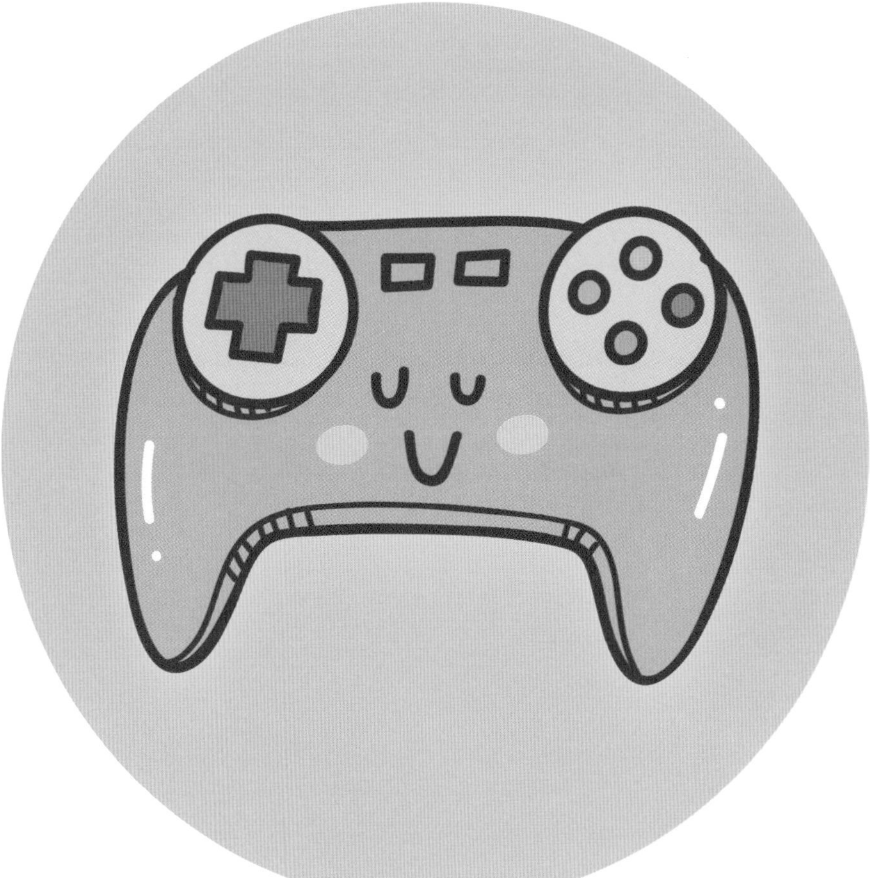

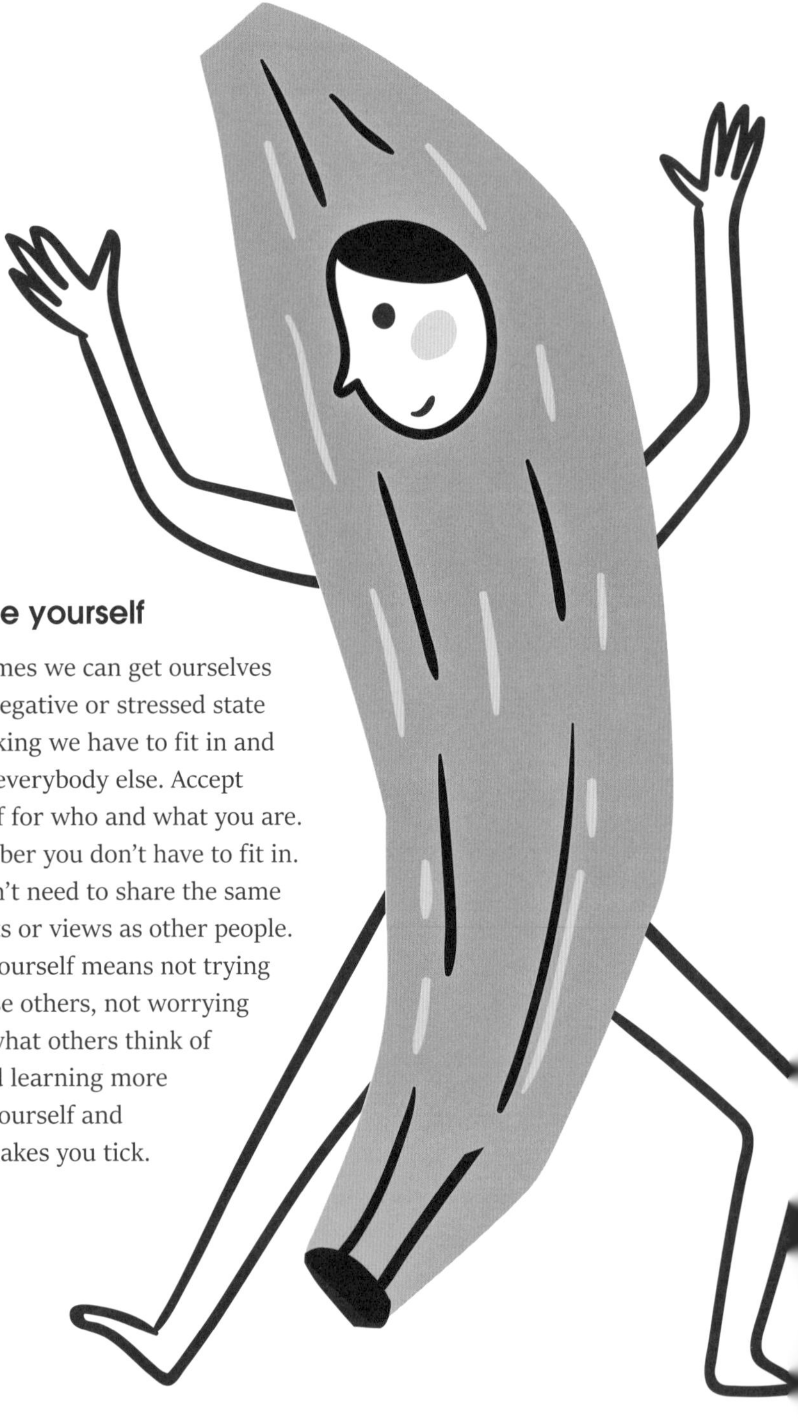

Just be yourself

Sometimes we can get ourselves into a negative or stressed state by thinking we have to fit in and be like everybody else. Accept yourself for who and what you are. Remember you don't have to fit in. You don't need to share the same interests or views as other people. Being yourself means not trying to please others, not worrying about what others think of you and learning more about yourself and what makes you tick.

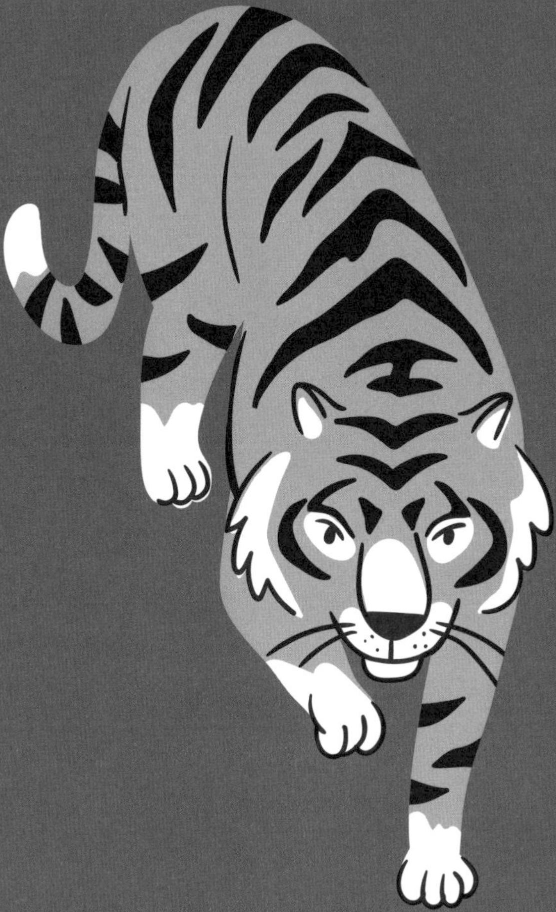

Fear is normal

Embrace fear rather than trying to overcome it. Accept that it's perfectly natural to be scared sometimes. High achievers and successful types aren't necessarily fearless – they embrace fear and accept that it's there, but they don't let it hold them back. Being scared or fearful means you're about to do something brave that's out of your comfort zone. Give yourself some credit.

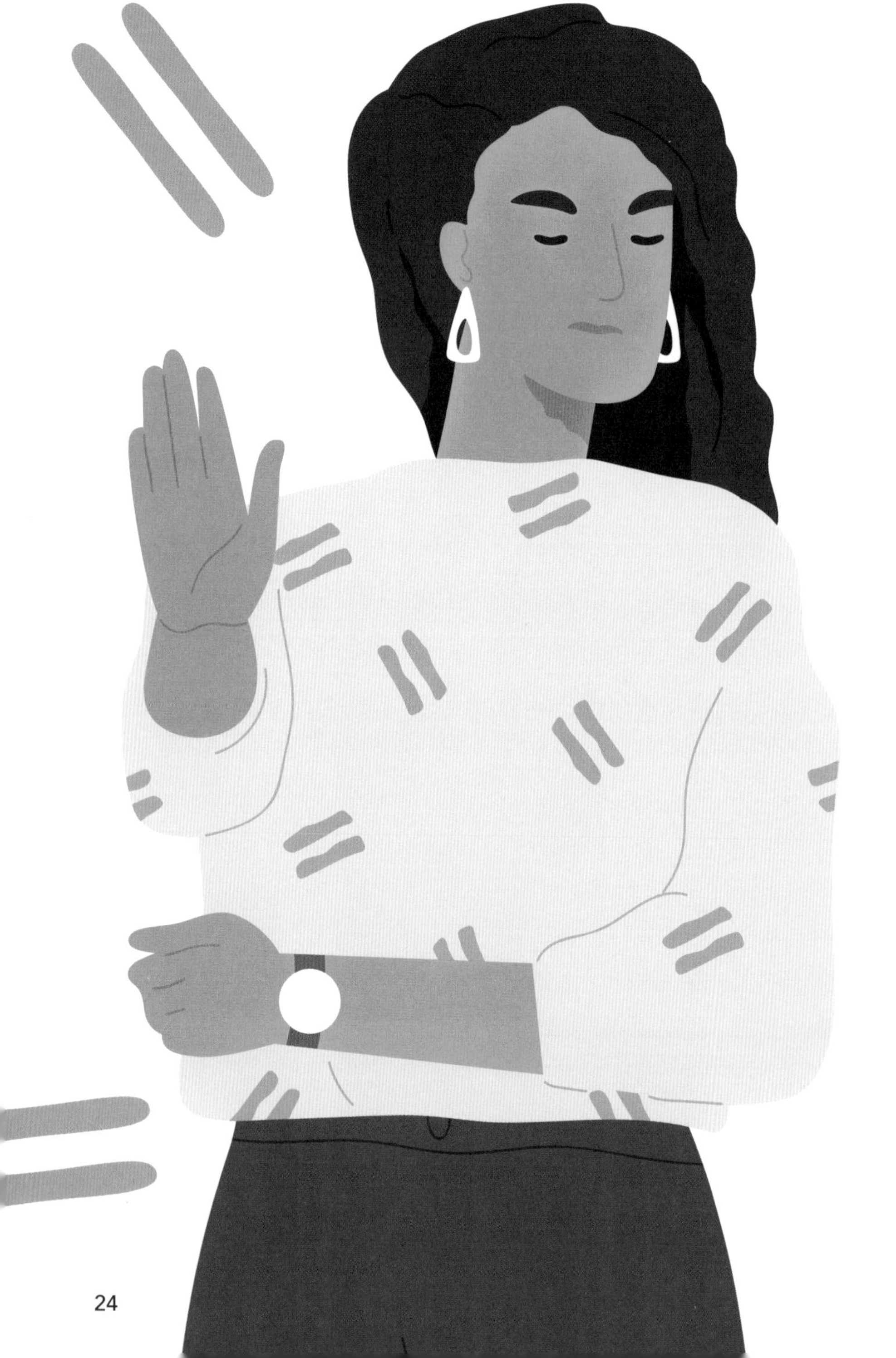

Know what you stand for

If you are constantly feeling anxious, unhappy or overwhelmed, it may be time to look at your values and beliefs and see if they are being compromised in any way. Your values are long-lasting beliefs about what is important to you. A belief is an idea that you hold as being true. An example of your beliefs being compromised might be that you are doing a job you don't like that goes against your moral or ethical principles, making you feel like you're putting on a mask and not being yourself when you're at work. Be true to your values and you will immediately feel your energy and sense of well-being increase.

One small positive thought in the morning can change your whole day

Recognize your limits

Constantly multi-tasking is likely to overwhelm your already busy mind. Instead of trying to get all of your to-do list done simultaneously and causing yourself unnecessary stress, make a short list of tasks to complete and focus on one at a time. If you're working, close your email inbox while you finish that report; put your phone on silent and avoid other digital distractions. Cross each task off a list as you go through them one by one. This will give you a sense of feeling in control again.

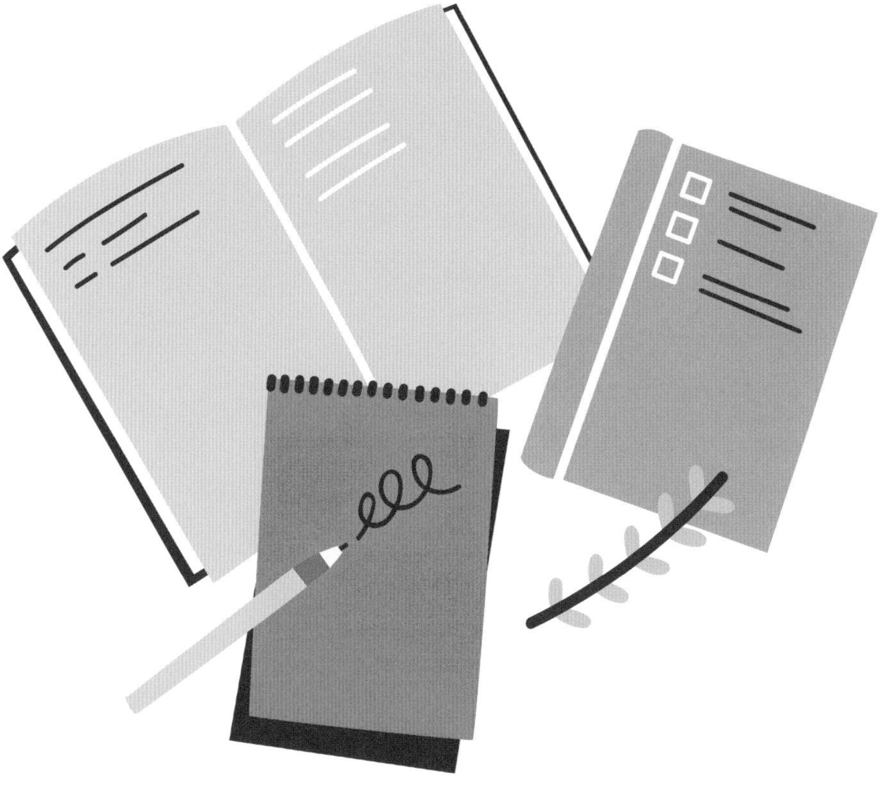

Why worry?
If you've done the
very best you can,
worrying won't make
it any better.

Walt Disney

It isn't where you come from, it's where you're going that counts

Challenge procrastination

Putting things off and leaving them until the last minute is a sure-fire way to raise your stress levels. Imagine a freelance journalist who has an article to write, due the next day; they know it needs to be done but they put it off and use other tasks to distract them from it, such as checking emails or doing housework. Before they know it, the day has gone and they still haven't put finger to keyboard. This may induce anxiety and cause their thoughts to spiral out of control, worrying that they will have to rush through it and compromise its quality – perhaps they become concerned that submitting a poorly written article will affect their reputation. In short, putting the task off until the eleventh hour caused the journalist anxiety that could have been avoided altogether. Don't leave tasks until the last minute or you risk putting yourself in stressful situations you could have prevented. When you complete the task you've been putting off, you'll feel a sense of relief. Do the thing that's making you uncomfortable or pushing you outside of your comfort zone. You'll feel better for it.

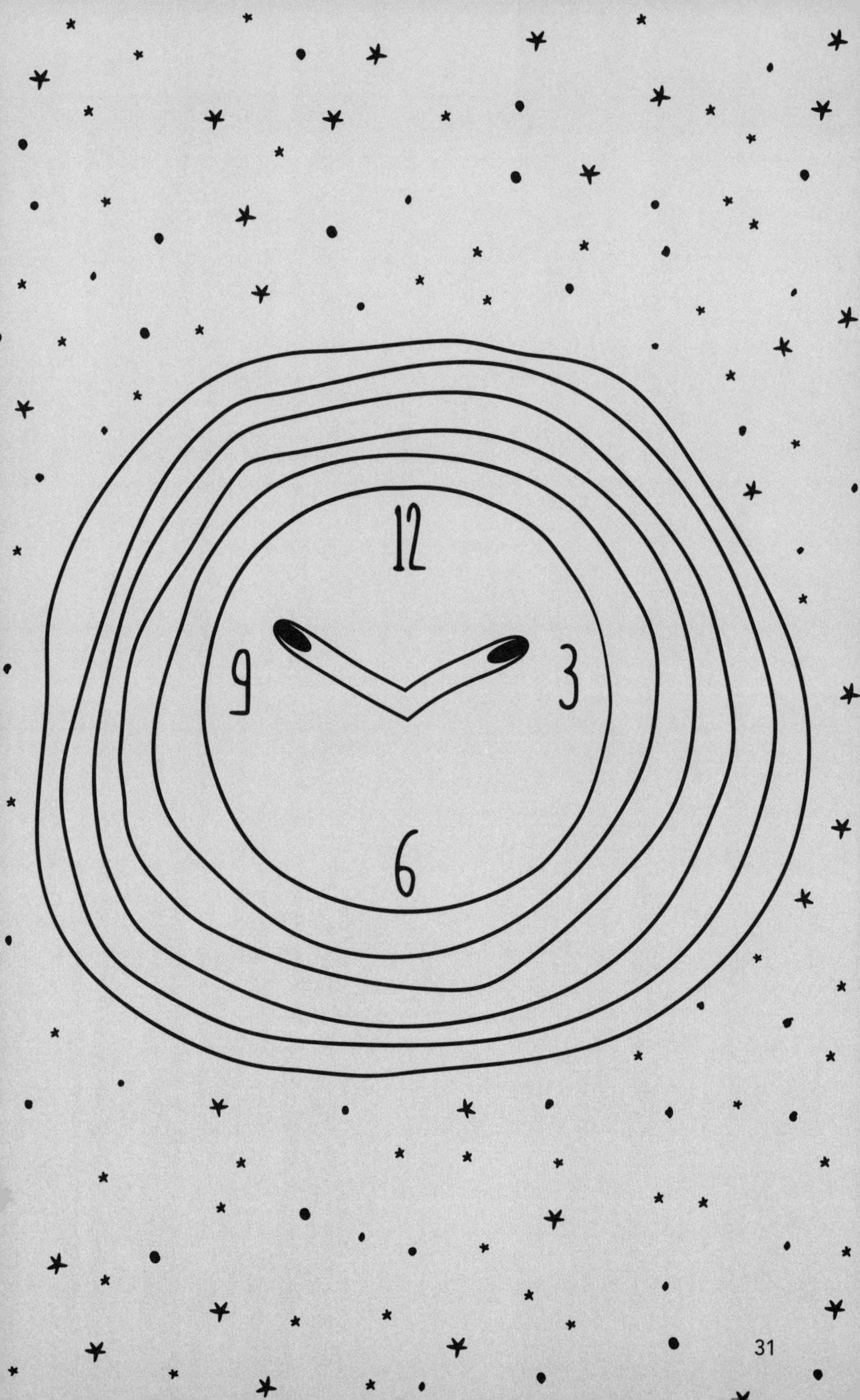
12
9
3
6

Ease the pressure

It's easy to worry or feel anxious if we put pressure on ourselves to do well, such as expecting that we will succeed at a new task or taking on a new job and being keen to make a good impression. Stay positive, but be realistic with your expectations. You can't always be good at something new straight away. Approach a new task or job with an open mind. Roll with the punches and you may find your new, relaxed attitude makes you better placed to complete the task and do it well, because you're focused and thinking more clearly.

Difficulties are just things to overcome after all.

Ernest Shackleton

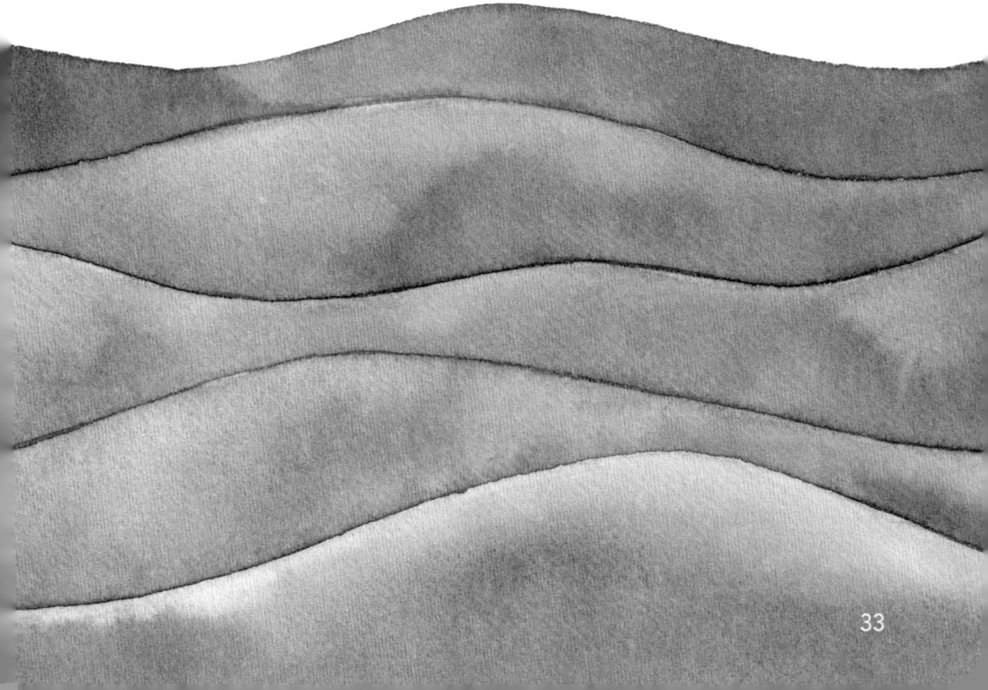

TRAIN YOUR MIND TO SEE THE GOOD IN EVERYTHING

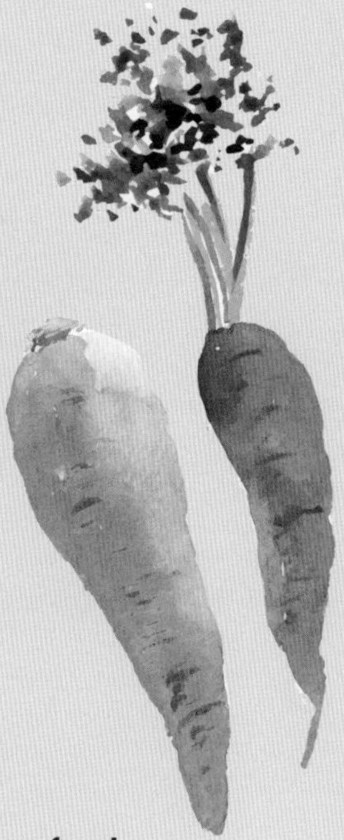

Perfectly imperfect

Don't strive for perfection. It's easy to worry too much about being faultless – whether that's having the perfect body or feeling like we have to be witty, intelligent and great company to our family and peers all the time. No one is perfect. The most accomplished and interesting people are those who have learned from their mistakes and imperfections. Be you, with all of your quirks and flaws. In an age where everyone feels pressure to conform and even look the same, your "imperfections" are what make you unique.

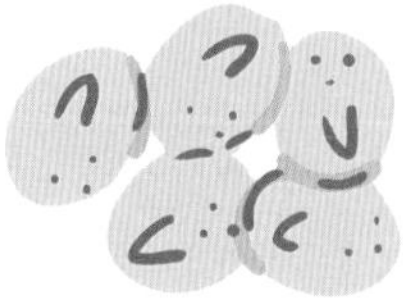

Appreciate your omegas

We know a healthy diet is good for our bodies, but it also has strong links to mental and emotional well-being, as well as the obvious physical benefits. One aspect of your diet that it is particularly important to focus on is omega-3 fatty acids, which are thought to be good for the function of a healthy central nervous system, improving brain function and concentration and in turn, boosting your mood. This is because omega-3 fatty acids can easily travel through brain cell membrane and interact with mood-related molecules. They also have anti-inflammatory actions which may help to relieve depression. A study published in the *Journal of Epidemiology and Community Health*, which analyzed 26 previously published studies involving over 150,000 participants, found that those who consumed the most fish were less likely to suffer from depression. Good sources of omega-3 fatty acids include salmon, sardines and mackerel; vegan sources include seaweed, chia seeds and flax seeds.

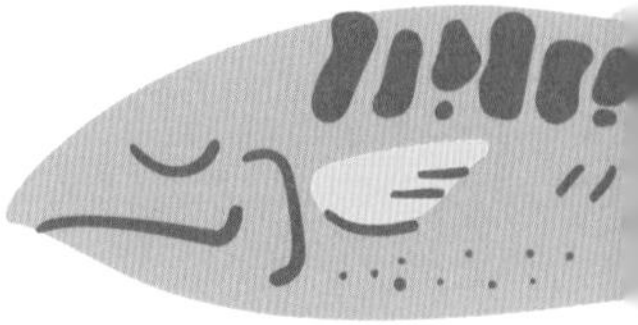

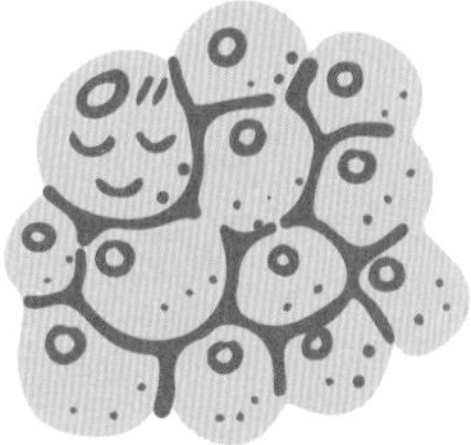

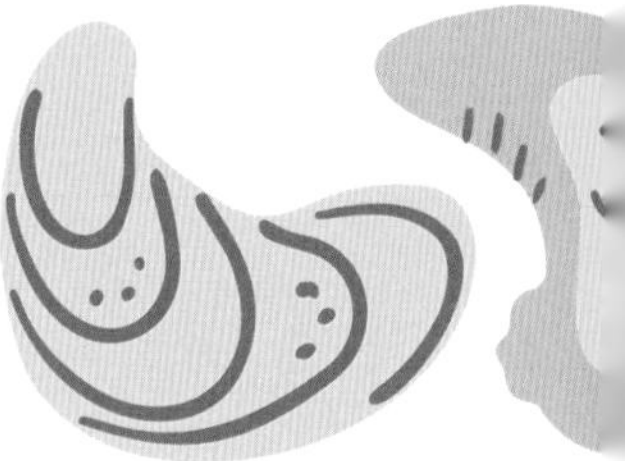

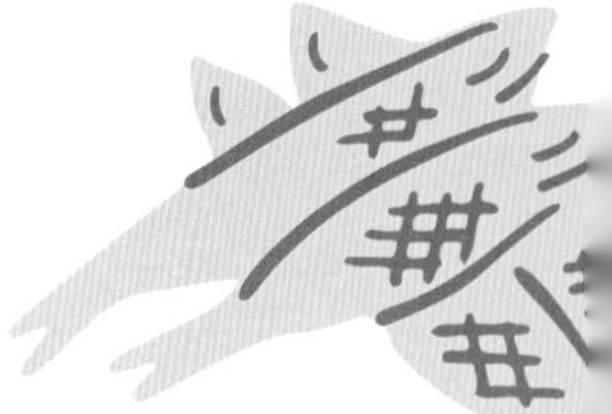

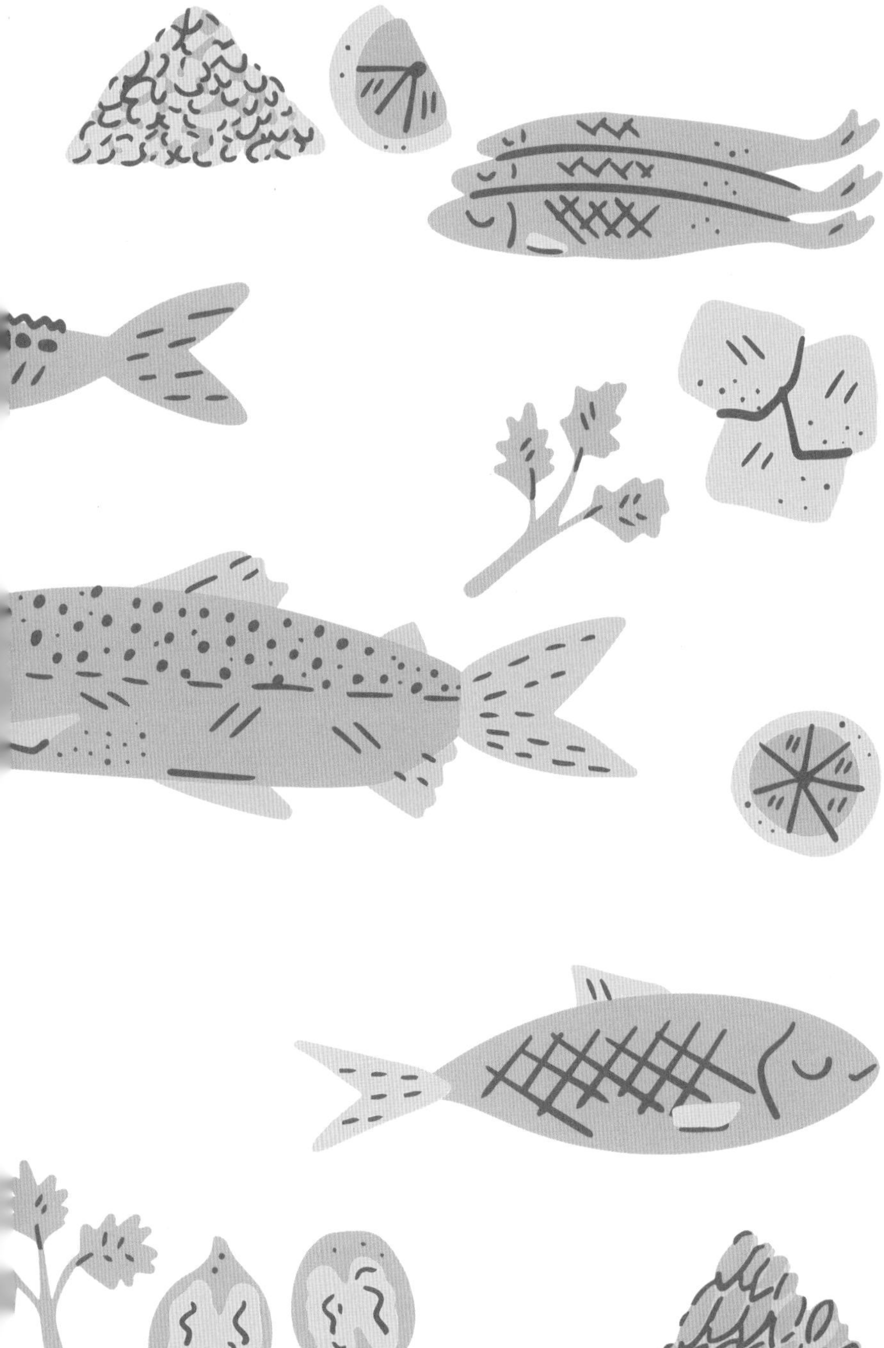

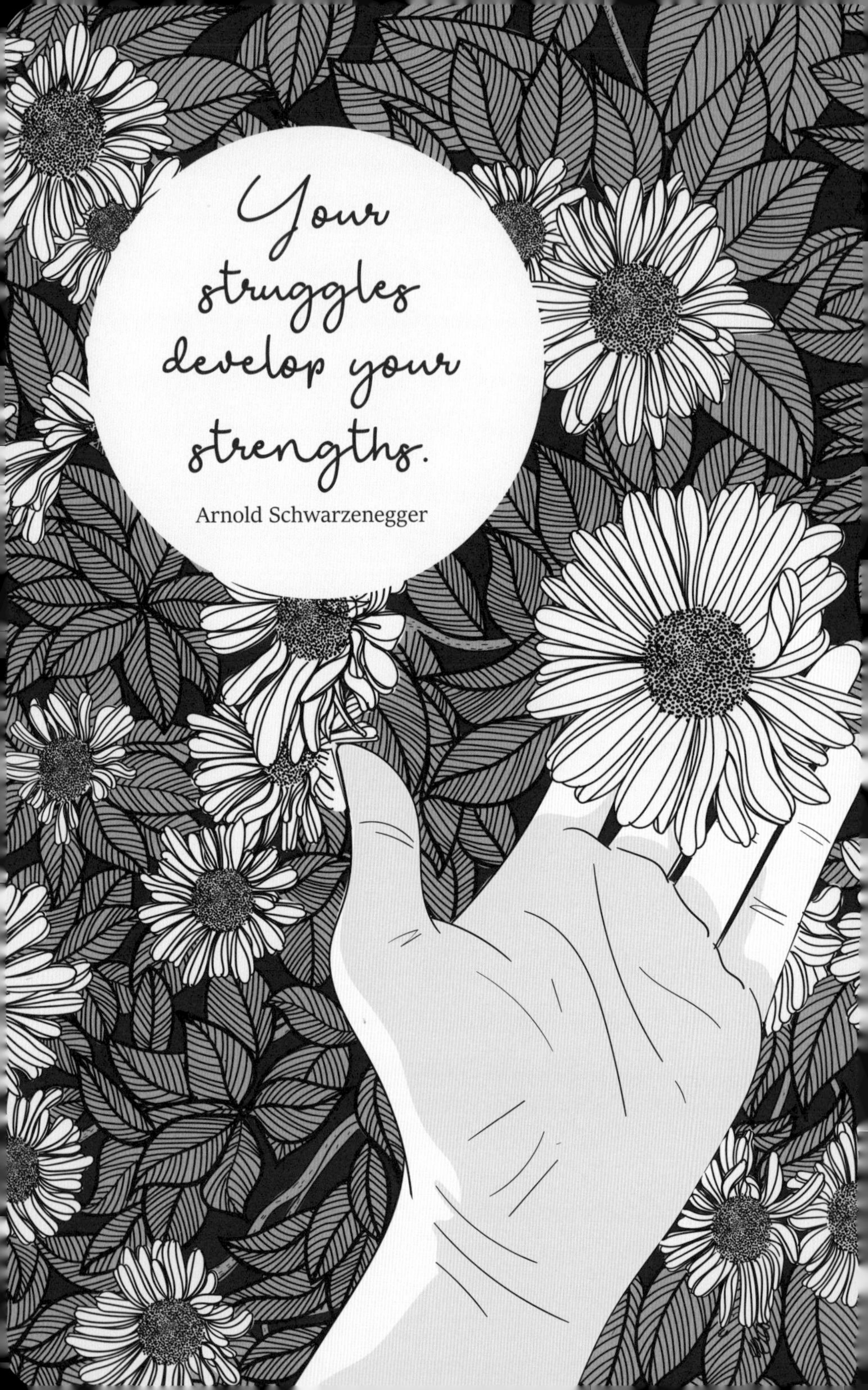
Your struggles develop your strengths.
Arnold Schwarzenegger

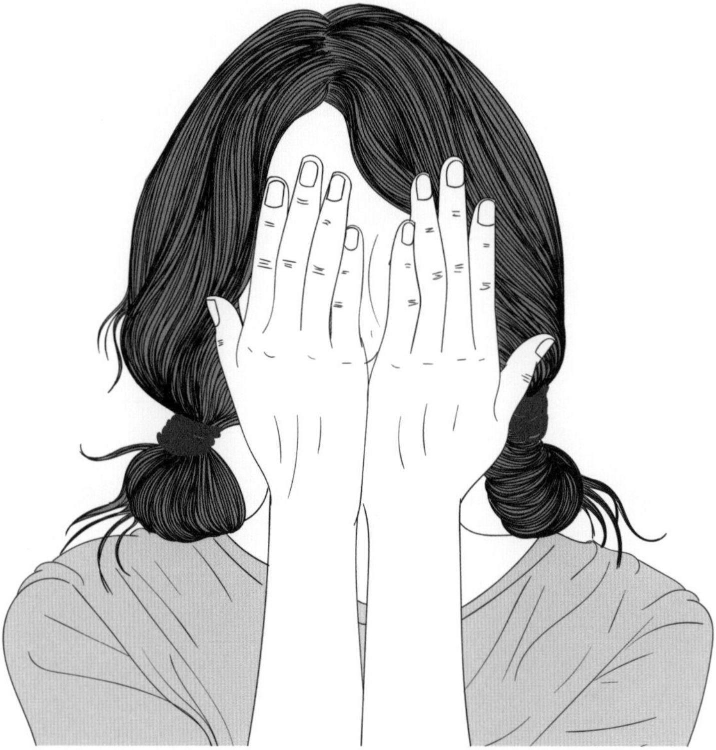

Be honest with yourself

If you are feeling anxious about a forthcoming situation, such as an event you have to attend, take a long hard look at it and work out what's causing your anxiety. Are you nervous because you feel self-conscious or awkward in social situations, or is it the people attending the event that you don't want to see? If you can be really honest with yourself about what's causing your worry, you may be able to address it beforehand – even if it's just to tell yourself you'll avoid certain people that cause you stress.

DON'T STRESS YOURSELF ABOUT THINGS

YOU CANNOT CONTROL OR CHANGE

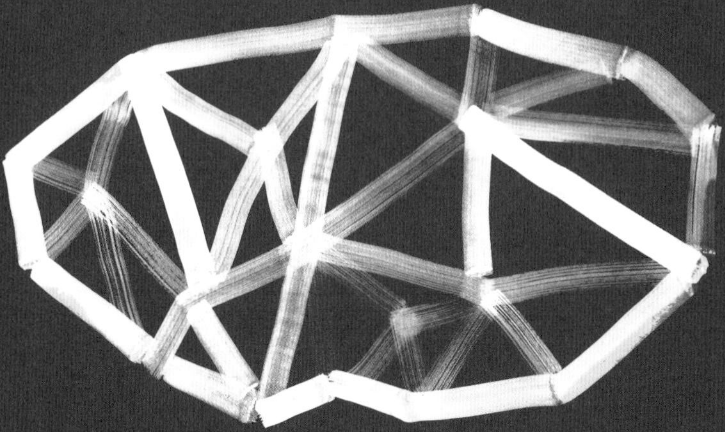

Don't overthink it

Try not to let your thoughts run away with you. Imagining the very worst possible scenario or outcome in a given situation is often referred to by psychologists as "catastrophizing". An example might be having a few harsh words with your partner and thinking you might break up because they've walked off, rather than understanding that they may simply need time to calm down before you can talk and resolve the problem. Letting your mind wander to what would happen if you were to break up – like where you would live and how you would feel about being on your own – is certain to raise anxiety levels.

Never let life's hardships disturb you... no one can avoid problems, not even saints or sages.

Nichiren

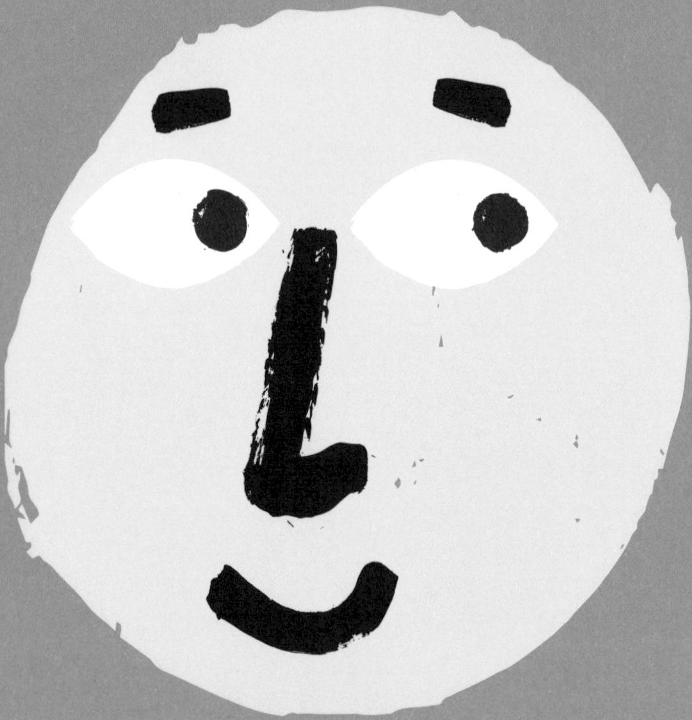

Manage stressful encounters

Stress can be caused by conflict with family members or close friends – especially at certain times of year when there's a holiday and you spend more time with relatives and loved ones than normal. If you are dealing with family stress or someone is annoying you, ask yourself how important

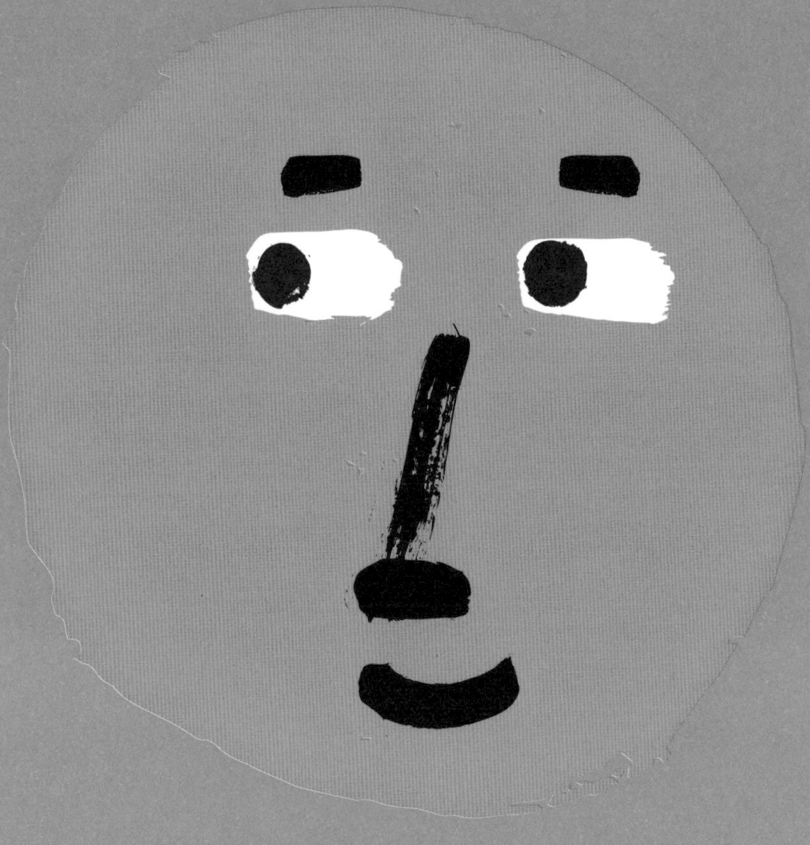

what they are saying or doing will be tomorrow. Will it matter? Remember that their views are just that – their views; you don't need to take them on board. Rising above unpleasant or cutting remarks says a lot about you and your ability to deal with stressful situations in a dignified way.

THERE IS

ALWAYS A

REASON

TO SMILE

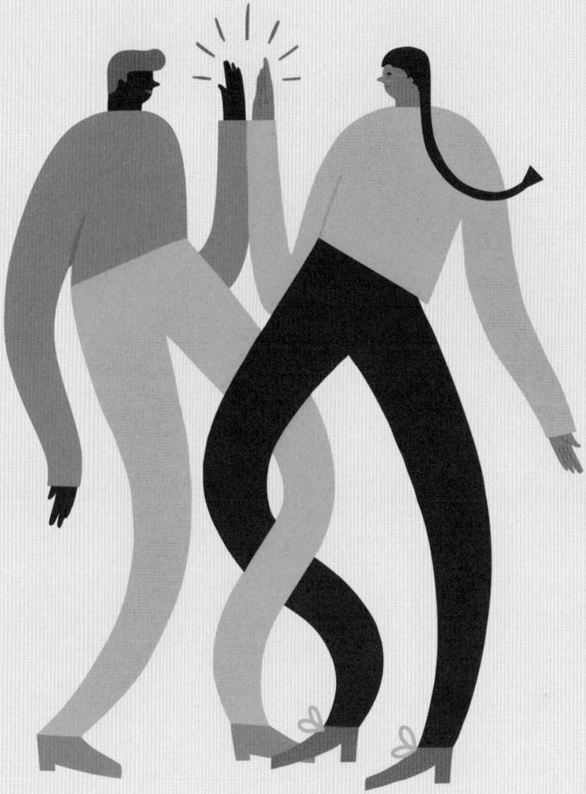

You are not alone

It may help to know that anxiety affects us all at different stages in our lives. You are definitely not alone and it's more common than many people realize. However, you can make a start on overcoming your anxiety. The next chapter explores several techniques you can use to change your mindset and improve your outlook, leaving you better placed to cope with stress and worry.

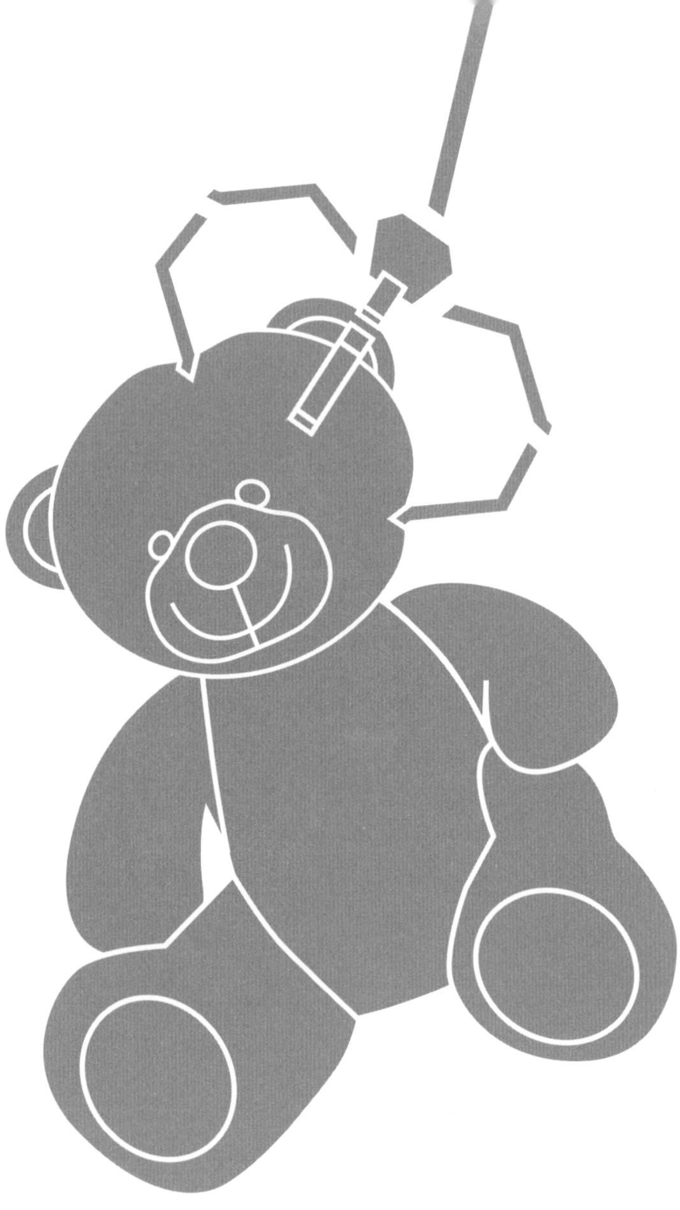

You don't have to control your thoughts. You just have to stop letting them control you.

Dan Millman

PART TWO:

BE KIND TO YOUR MIND

Other people may have told you to stop worrying, helpfully pointing out that worry won't change anything. However, even though anxiety itself might seem unavoidable, it can be controlled, and self-awareness is key.

Your mind is like a computer: if you programme it well, it will serve you well and work in your favour. This chapter explores how to manage your mindset and change your perceptions around feeling anxious, so that you can be more positive and resilient when problems or stressful situations may arise.

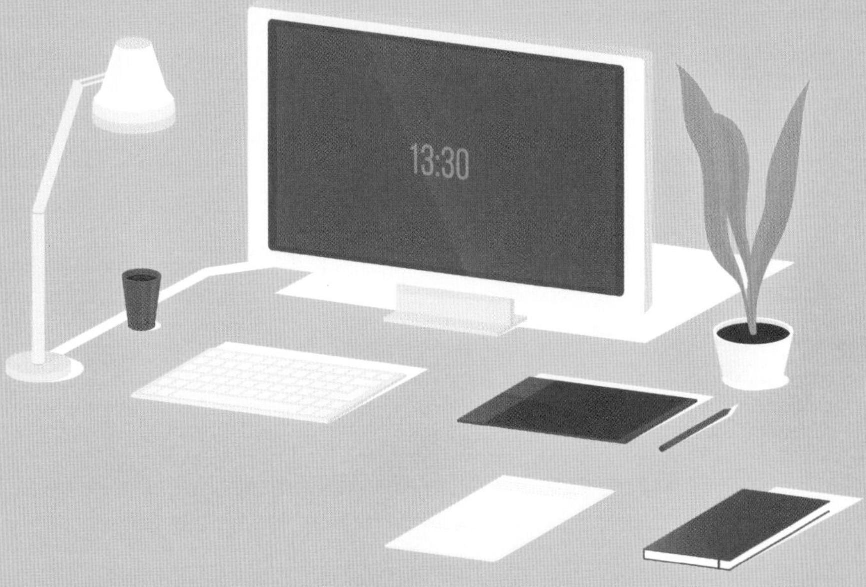

What's the very worst?

If you are worrying about something, ask yourself: what is the worst that could happen? Then work out what you could do if "the very worst" did happen. For instance, if you want to start a new business but you're worried that leaving your job will expose you to financial risk, look at the worst-case scenario. Maybe you'd have to find another job if your business idea didn't take off. Remind yourself that you have enough skill and experience to do that if you had to, so why worry?

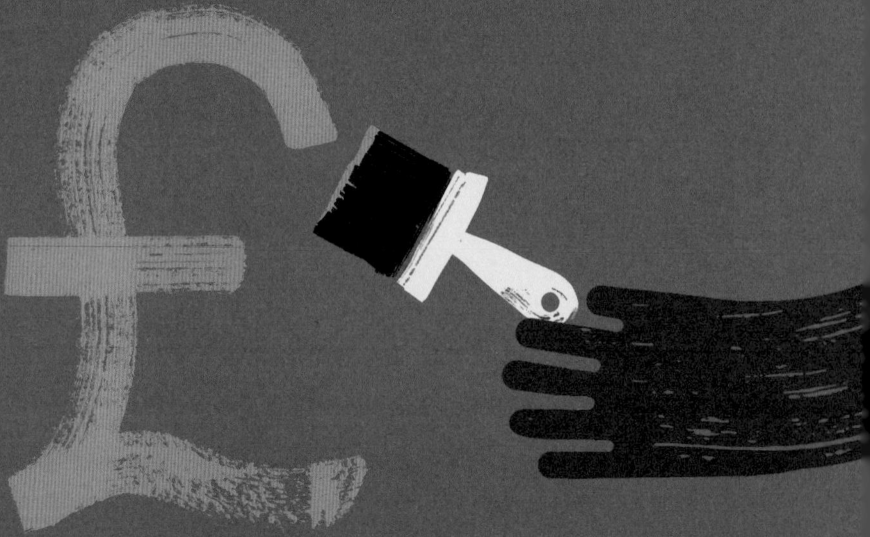

OVERTHINKING KEEPS YOU BUSY BUT TAKES YOU NOWHERE

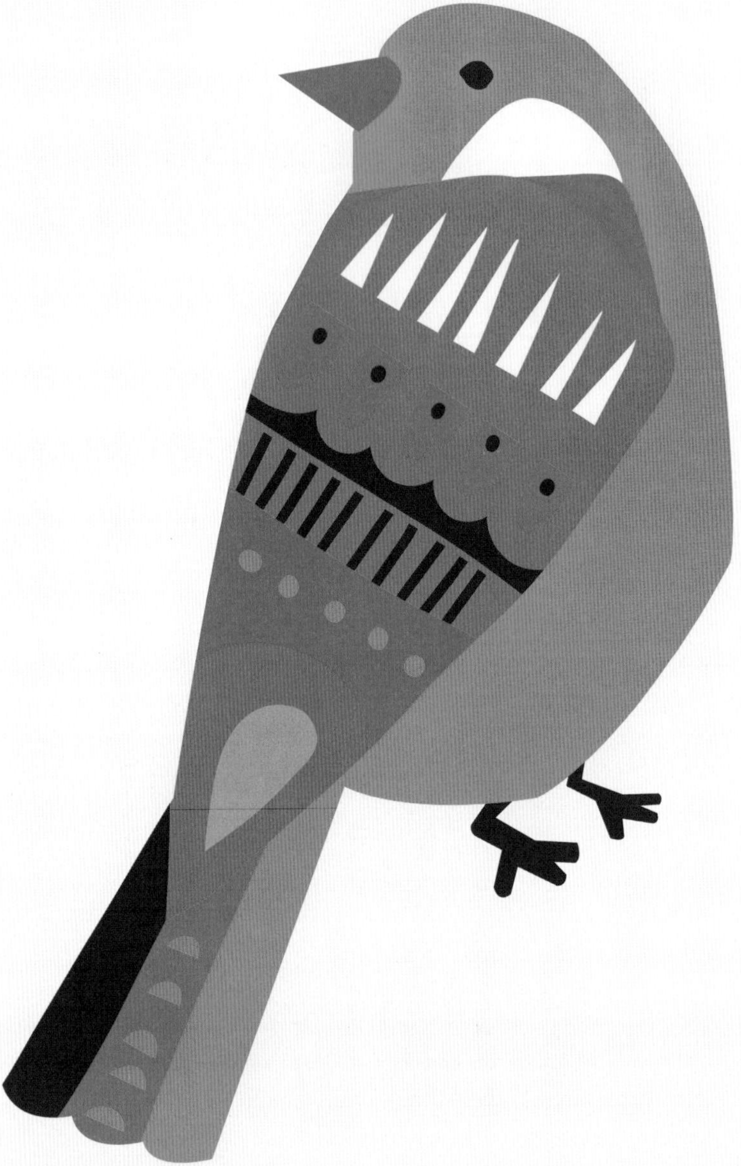

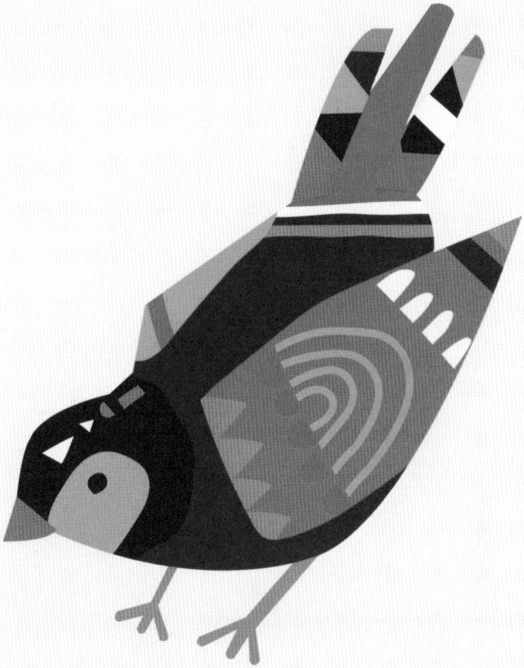

Avoid comparisons

You may look at your friends and peers and think they have it all sorted. They may appear to be happy, fulfilled and supported by their partner or family, but in reality they may be going through some difficult times or dealing with issues you're not even aware of. This tendency toward comparison with others is often exacerbated by our use of social media. While social media is a great tool for communication, it can also lead us to think that the "highlight reels" of our friends are representative of their lives as a whole. If ever you feel yourself looking at the "Insta story" or Facebook post of a friend and wondering why your life isn't as exciting as theirs and their friends', take a step back and remember that you are seeing something that they have created – not their day-to-day reality. Our lives can seem more challenging and difficult when we think everyone else has got the balance right. Remember that things aren't always what they seem.

Smile, breathe and go slowly.

Thích Nhất Hạnh

Interrupt anxiety with gratitude

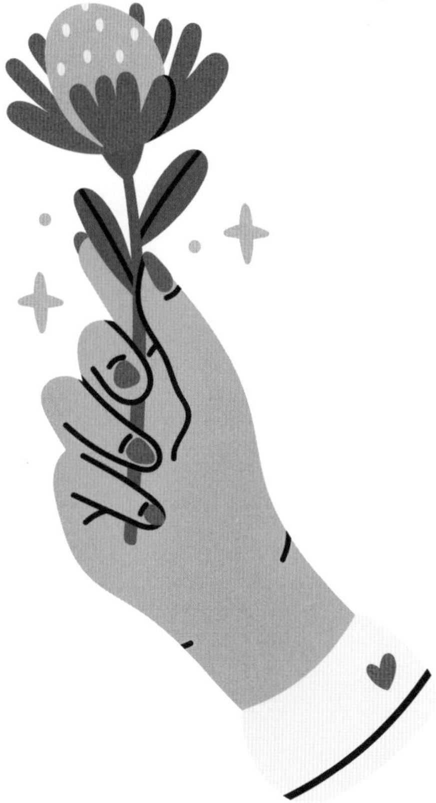

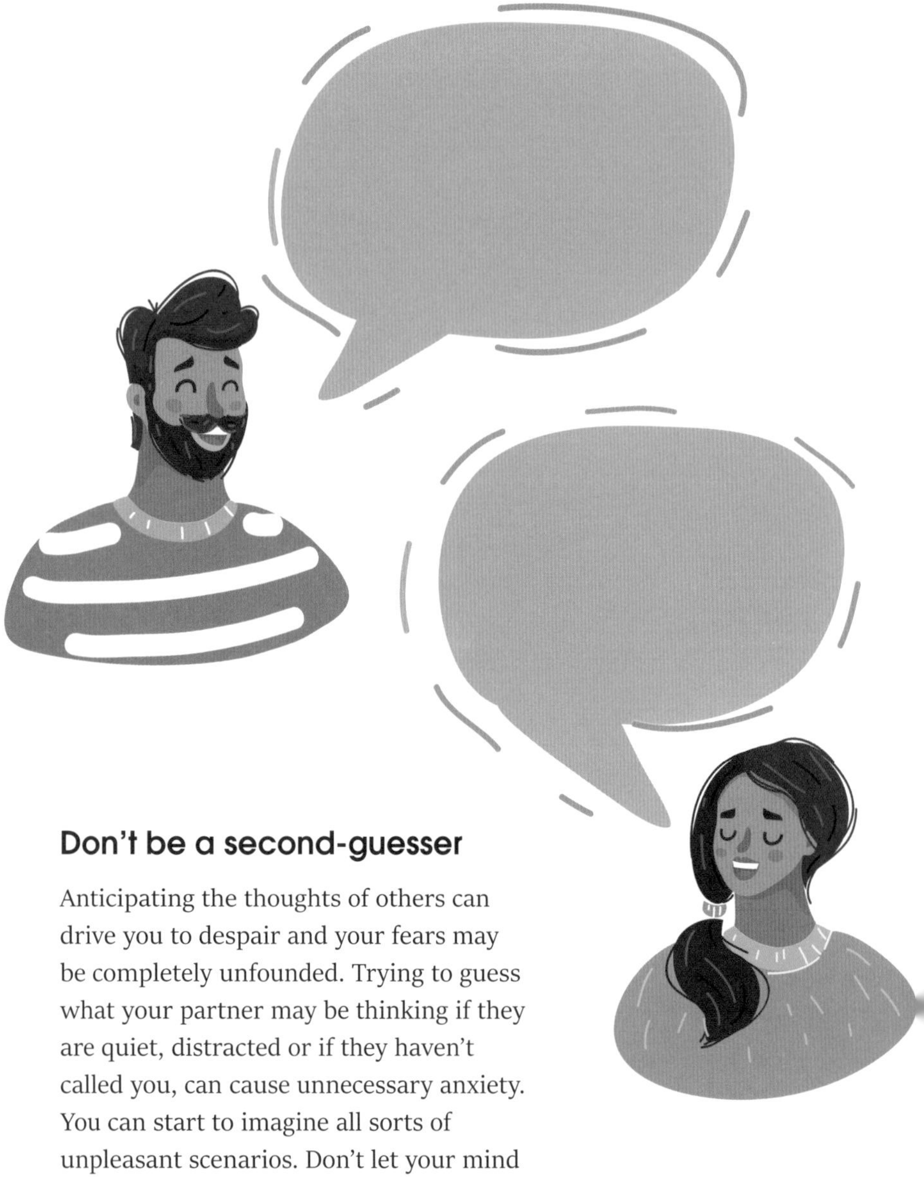

Don't be a second-guesser

Anticipating the thoughts of others can drive you to despair and your fears may be completely unfounded. Trying to guess what your partner may be thinking if they are quiet, distracted or if they haven't called you, can cause unnecessary anxiety. You can start to imagine all sorts of unpleasant scenarios. Don't let your mind run away with you. If you are worried about someone's mood or behaviour, communicate with them. Ask them what you want to ask rather than second-guessing and creating scenarios in your head that may not exist.

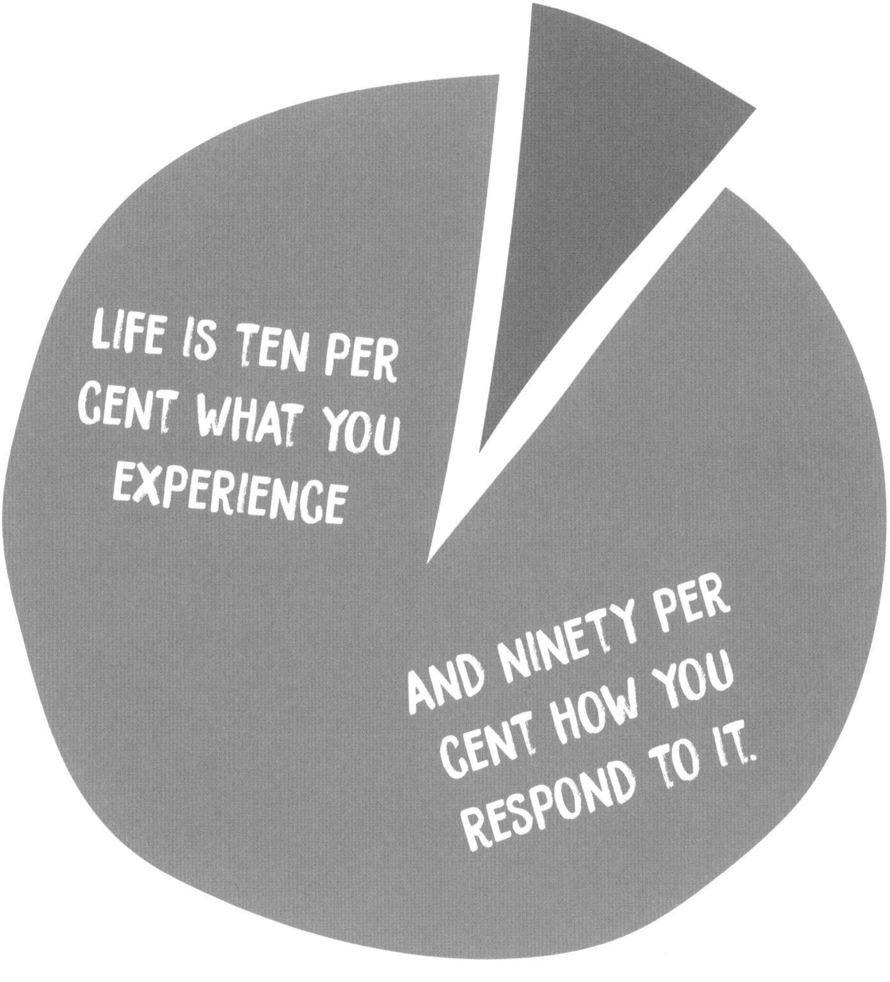

Charles R. Swindoll

Try not to problem-solve at night

Problems or issues can be amplified at night-time. If you're lying awake and it feels like everyone else is asleep, you may feel lonely and isolated – this isn't the best time to solve your problems or sort your life out. We usually sleep in cycles of 90 minutes to 2 hours, and it's normal to wake up and change position and then go back into the next stage of sleep. This behaviour benefitted early humans and kept us safe, as we could wake up and check for danger in the form of predators. Some of us wake up in between sleep cycles and have anxious thoughts. Mindfulness may help to reduce anxiety at night, or you may find that having a 20-minute "worry window" at least 4 hours before you go to bed, where you write down your worries and how you will deal with them, will clear your mind and help you sleep better.

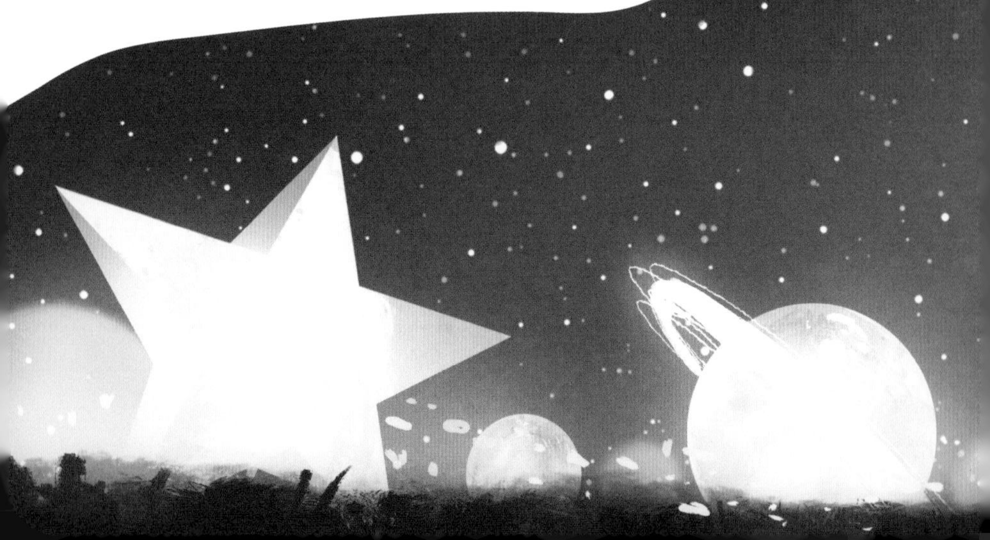

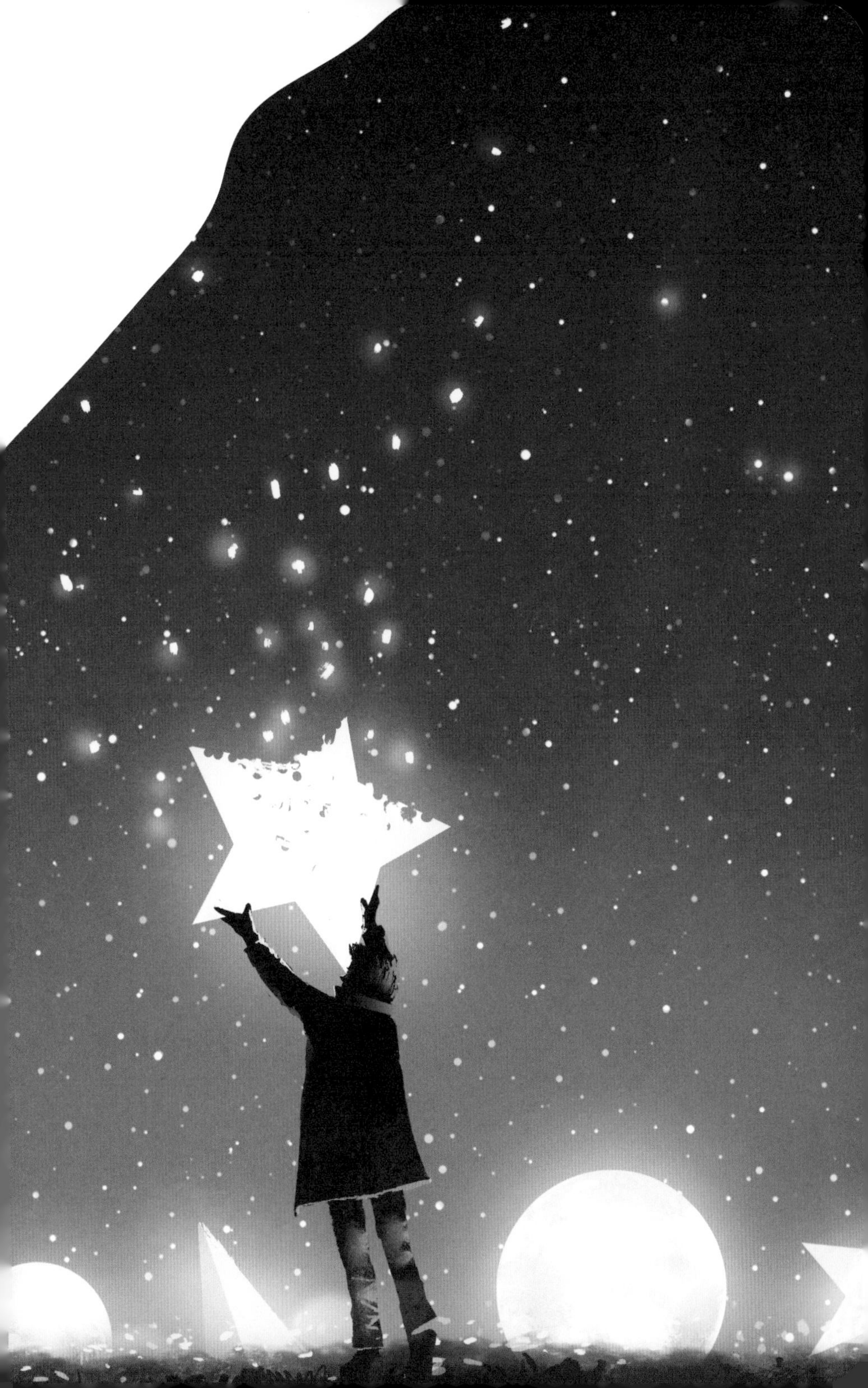

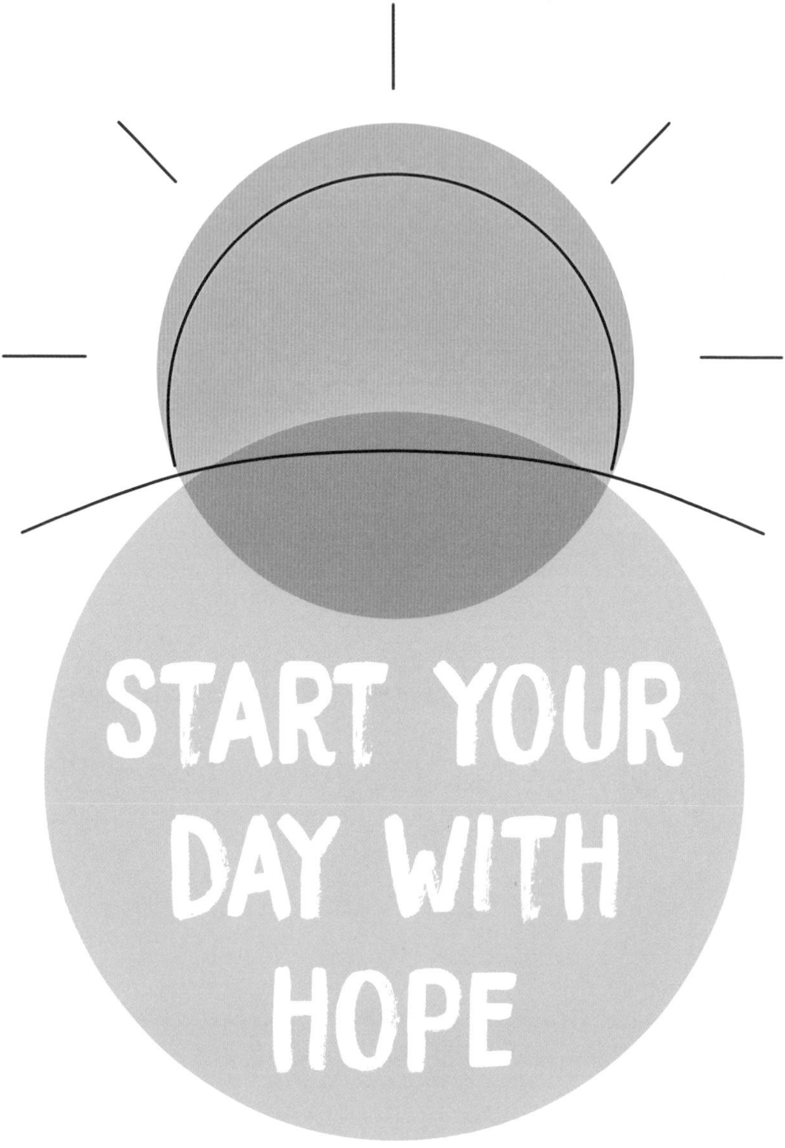
START YOUR
DAY WITH
HOPE

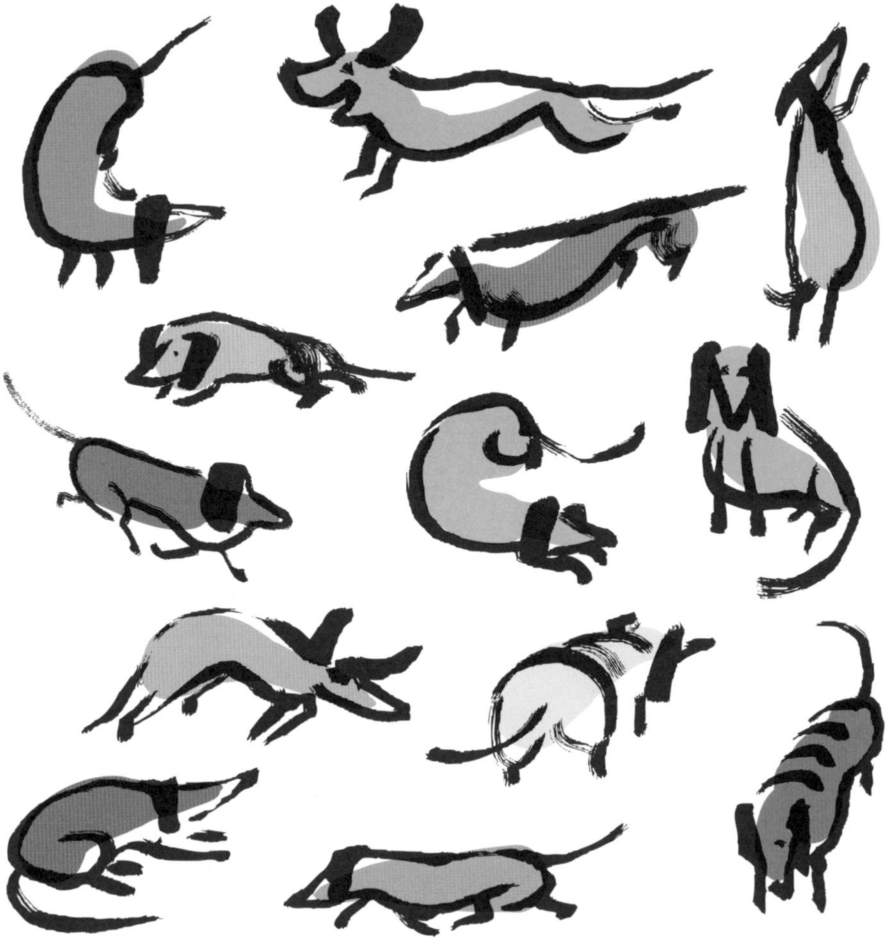

Trust your instincts

If you are trying to solve a problem or make a decision, and your mind is busy, tune in to what your gut is telling you. Anxiety is a frantic emotion, whereas intuition comes from a calm place. Listen to and trust your gut and you'll be more confident in your decisions.

YOUR MISSION:

BE SO BUSY
LOVING YOUR LIFE
THAT YOU HAVE NO
TIME FOR HATE,
REGRET OR FEAR.

Karen Salmansohn

Set a goal and be inspired

There's no better way to banish worry and anxiety than to find your purpose and focus on achieving a goal that means something to you. Find a role model. Think of someone (either someone famous or someone you know) who has turned their life around. Oprah Winfrey overcame a traumatic childhood to become one of America's top talk show hosts and TV producers. Lady Gaga was told by her former boyfriend she would never succeed, but beat numerous obstacles to become a top singer, songwriter and actress. Author J. K. Rowling had her books rejected by a dozen major publishing houses before she secured a publishing deal for her first book. If you feel that life is hopeless, difficult and never likely to change, think about what other people have achieved against the odds, purely because they have refused to give up. It's never too late to change and lead a better life.

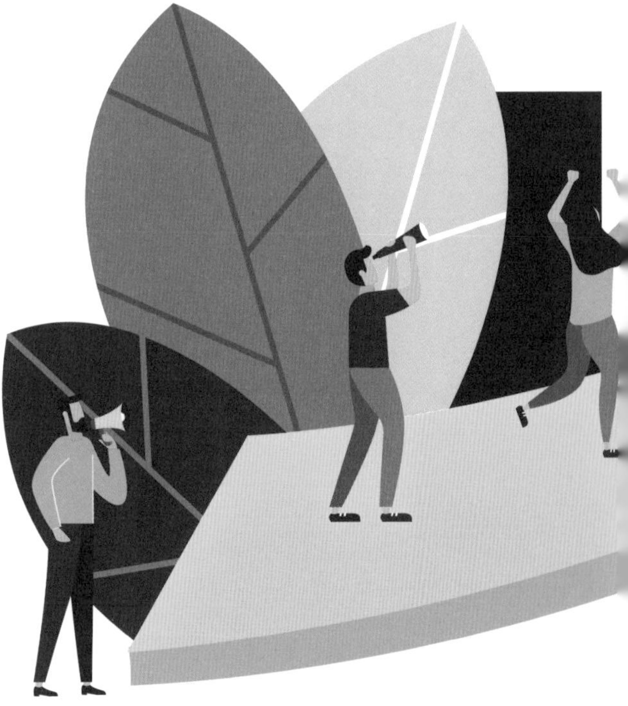

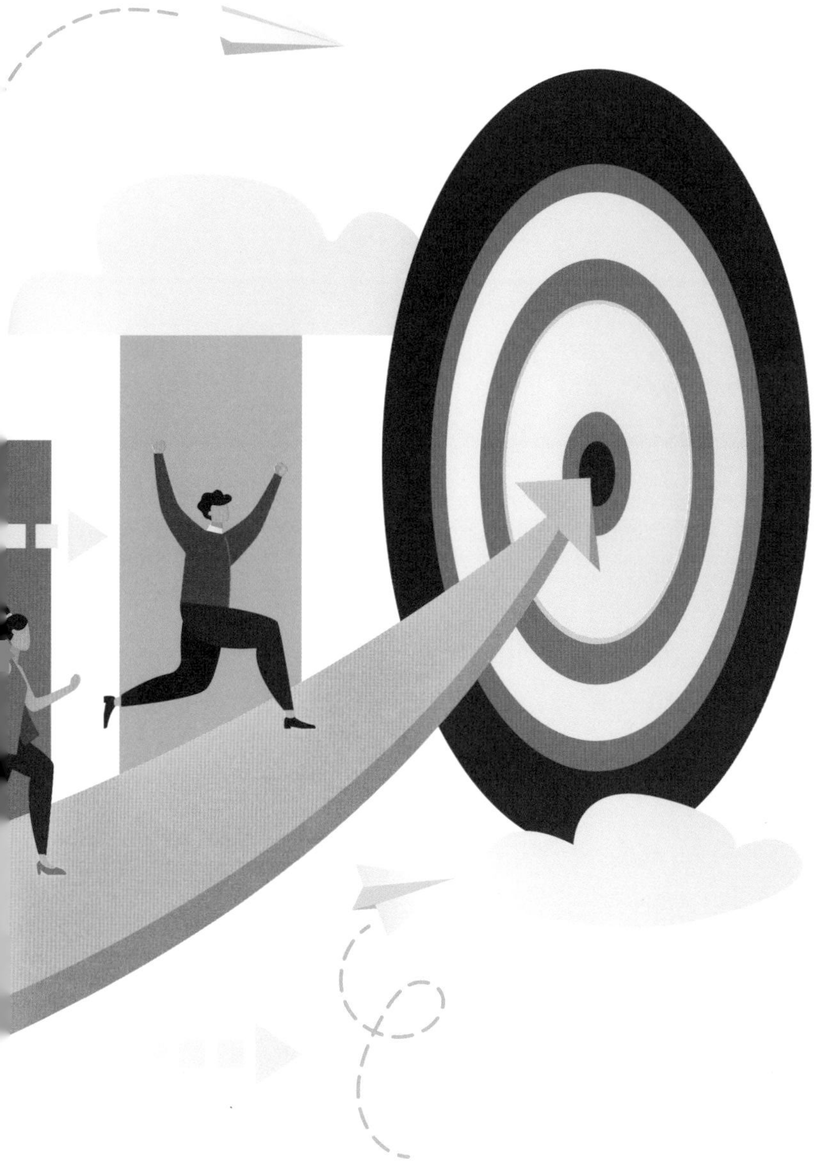

Move on

Learn from the past, but don't dwell on it and don't keep reliving things that went wrong or you feel you could have handled differently. Accept certain events as life lessons and move on. If you live in the past, you risk missing out on enjoying the present and moving forward in the future.

An obstacle
is often
a stepping
stone

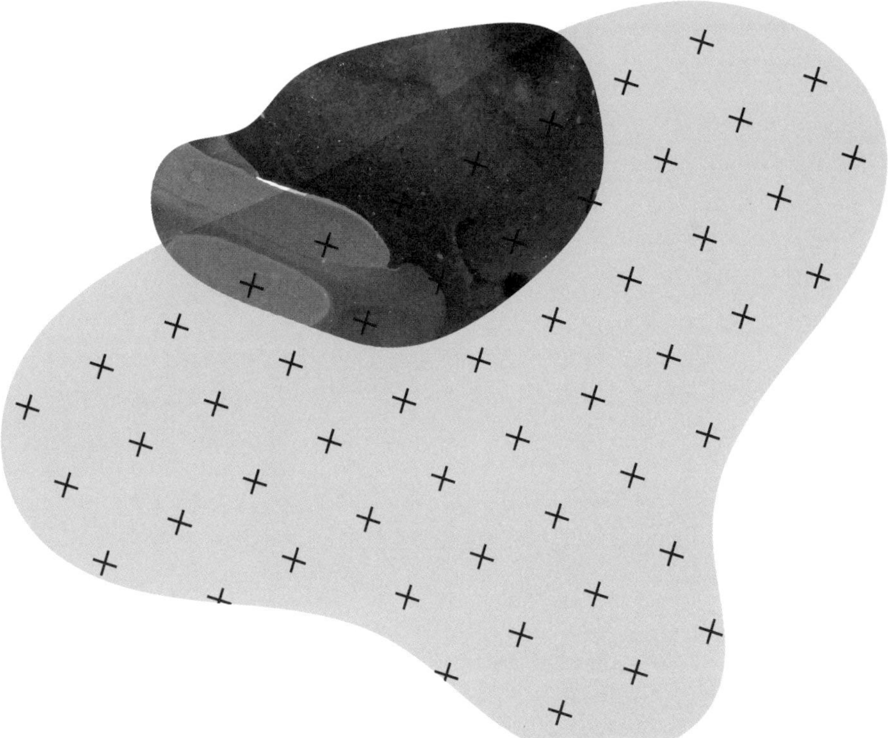

ANXIETY DOES NOT EMPTY TOMORROW OF ITS SORROWS, BUT ONLY EMPTIES TODAY OF ITS STRENGTH.

Charles Spurgeon

Take a digital detox

Learn how to switch off from digital distractions. It's common to feel anxious when our email inbox tells us we have another ten messages to read, or when we see a string of unread messages on WhatsApp. Have some time away from the noisy online world. If you go out for a walk, leave your phone at home; if you work out in the gym, leave your phone in the locker. Give yourself a break.

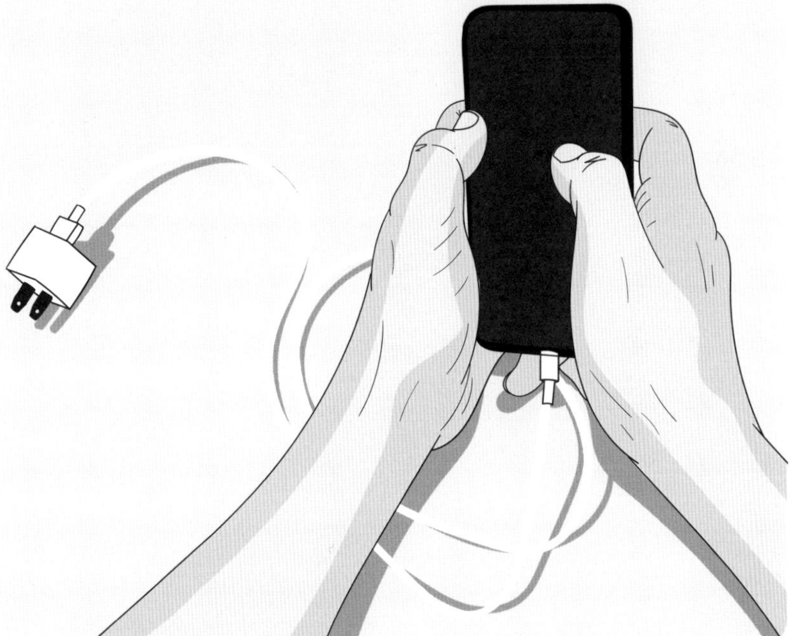

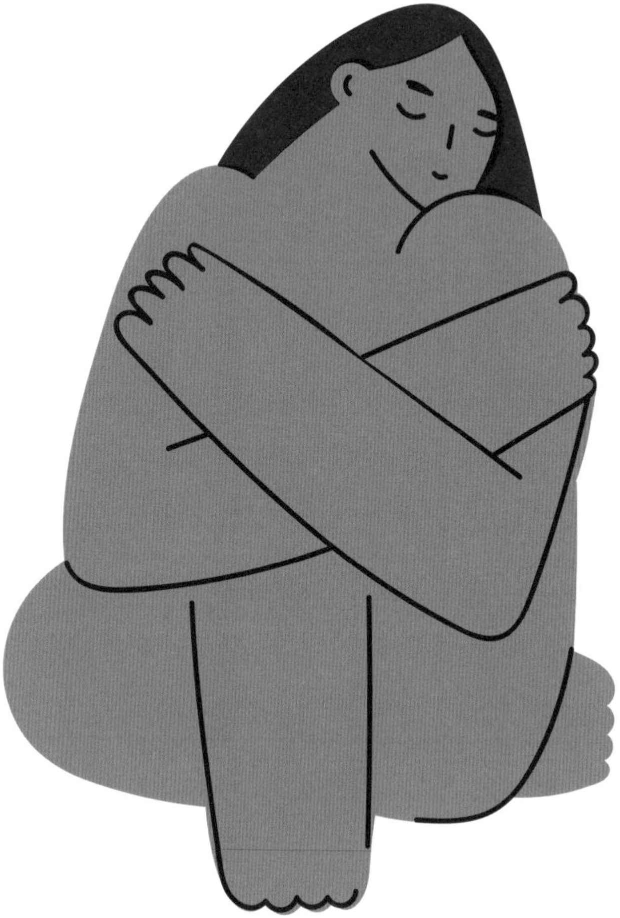

Change your view of you

Work on improving your perception of you. As the saying goes, you are the best project you'll ever work on. Change how you talk to yourself and retrain your brain to applaud the positive things you do, rather than focusing on things that go wrong. Be your own best friend.

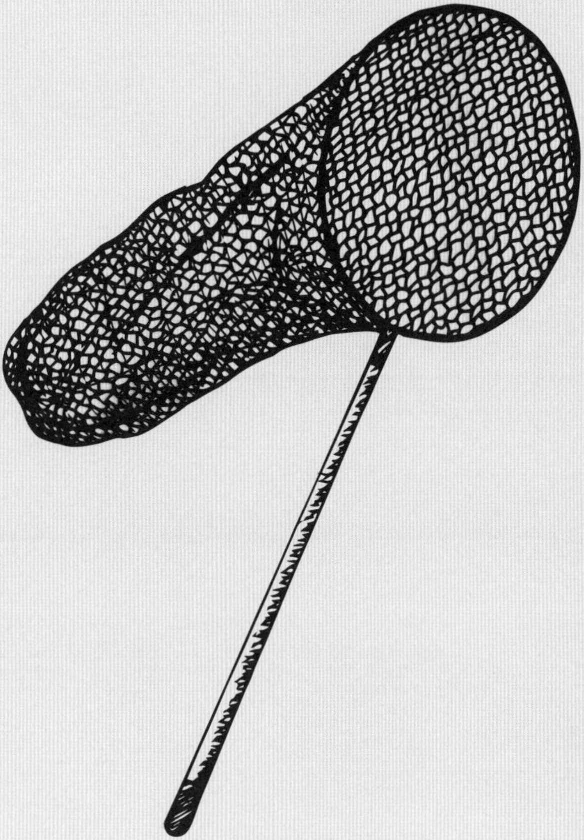

Attitudes are contagious.
Make yours worth catching.

Put a spotlight on your sleep

Even partial sleep deprivation can affect your mood. The World Health Organization recommends we get around 8 hours a night. According to *Harvard Health Publishing*, there is a close link between sleep and mental health. In one longitudinal study, conducted in a Michigan health maintenance organization, it was shown that those who reported a history of insomnia were four times more likely to develop major depression by the time they were interviewed again three years later.

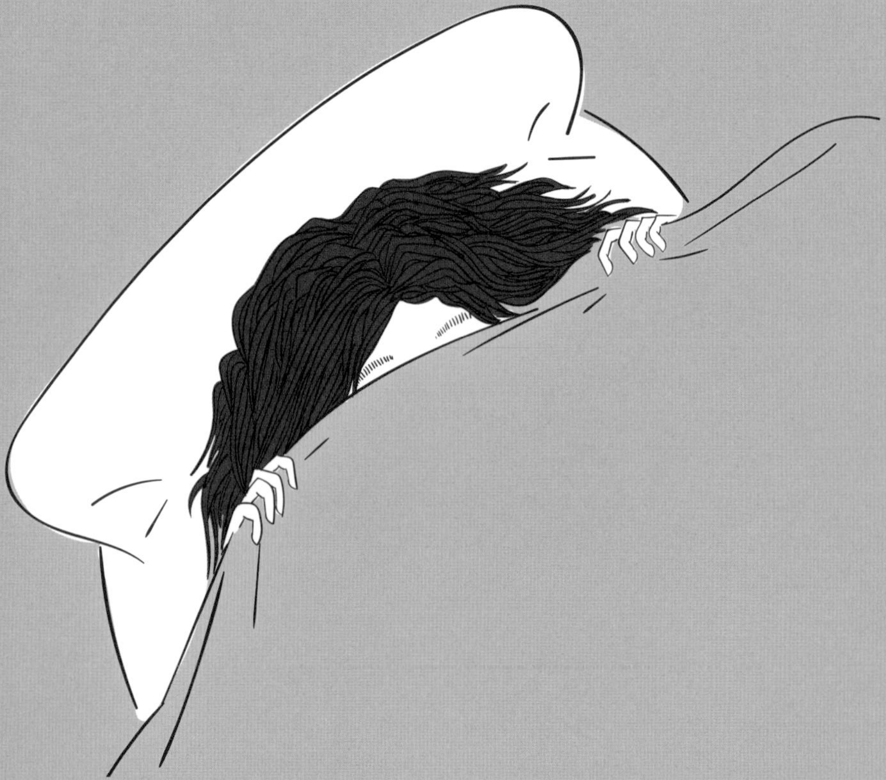

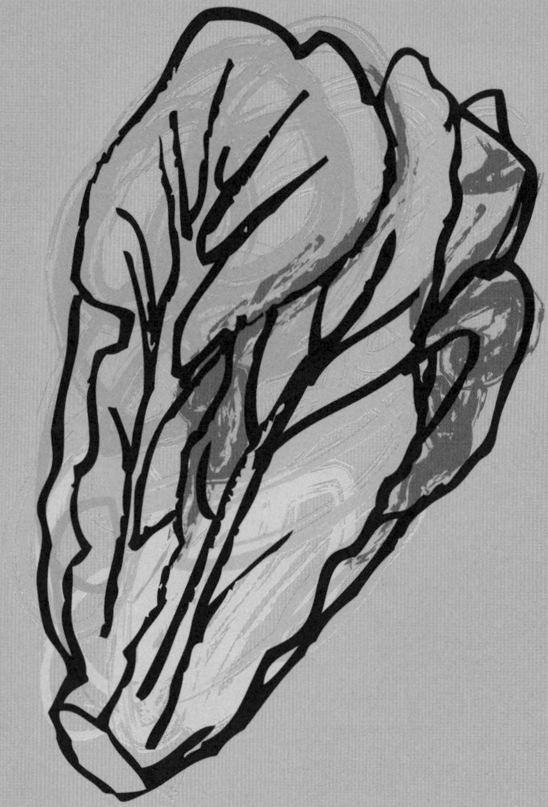

Try to establish a bedtime routine. Avoid checking emails or doing anything work related just before bed, as this will make your mind more alert and may increase anxiety. Go to bed at the same time each night, make sure you don't have phones near your bed so there are no charging lights to disturb you and make your room as dark as possible. Magnesium can help you sleep, which is available in plenty of food sources such as green leafy veg, fruits, nuts and seeds. If you struggle to get enough in your diet, you can also take it in the form of a supplement.

THEY ALWAYS SAY TIME CHANGES THINGS, BUT YOU ACTUALLY HAVE TO CHANGE THEM YOURSELF.

Andy Warhol

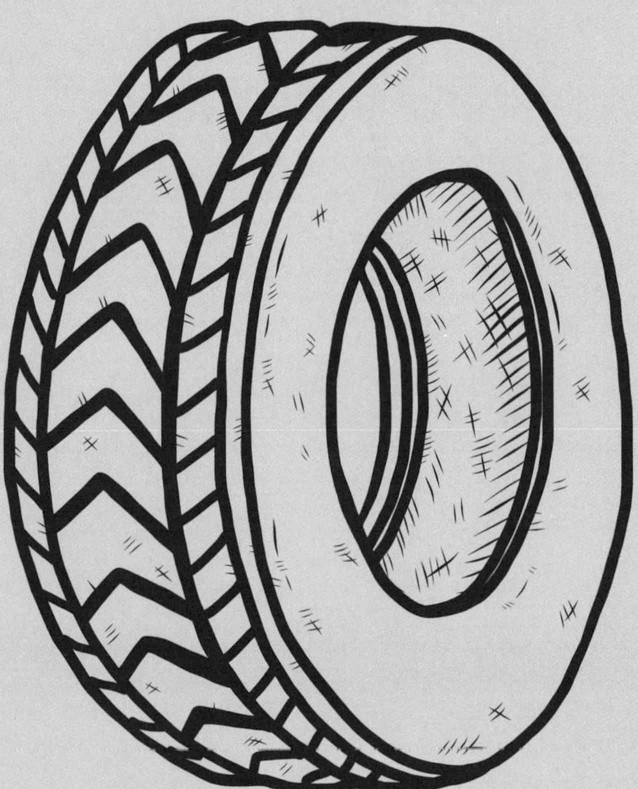

Don't believe everything you think

Act as if what you do makes a difference – it does.

William James

Don't let the past control you

If you want to feel more confident and let go of anxiety relating to your past, don't confuse your memory with facts. We all remember things differently and our brains store information that aligns with our values and beliefs. Your memory will not always be giving you accurate information about what happened. So, if something in your past is causing you worry or holding you back, revisit the facts related to a self-limiting belief and try to see it objectively; it may help you gain a more balanced perspective and enable you to move forward.

If you don't like something, change it. If you can't change it, change your attitude

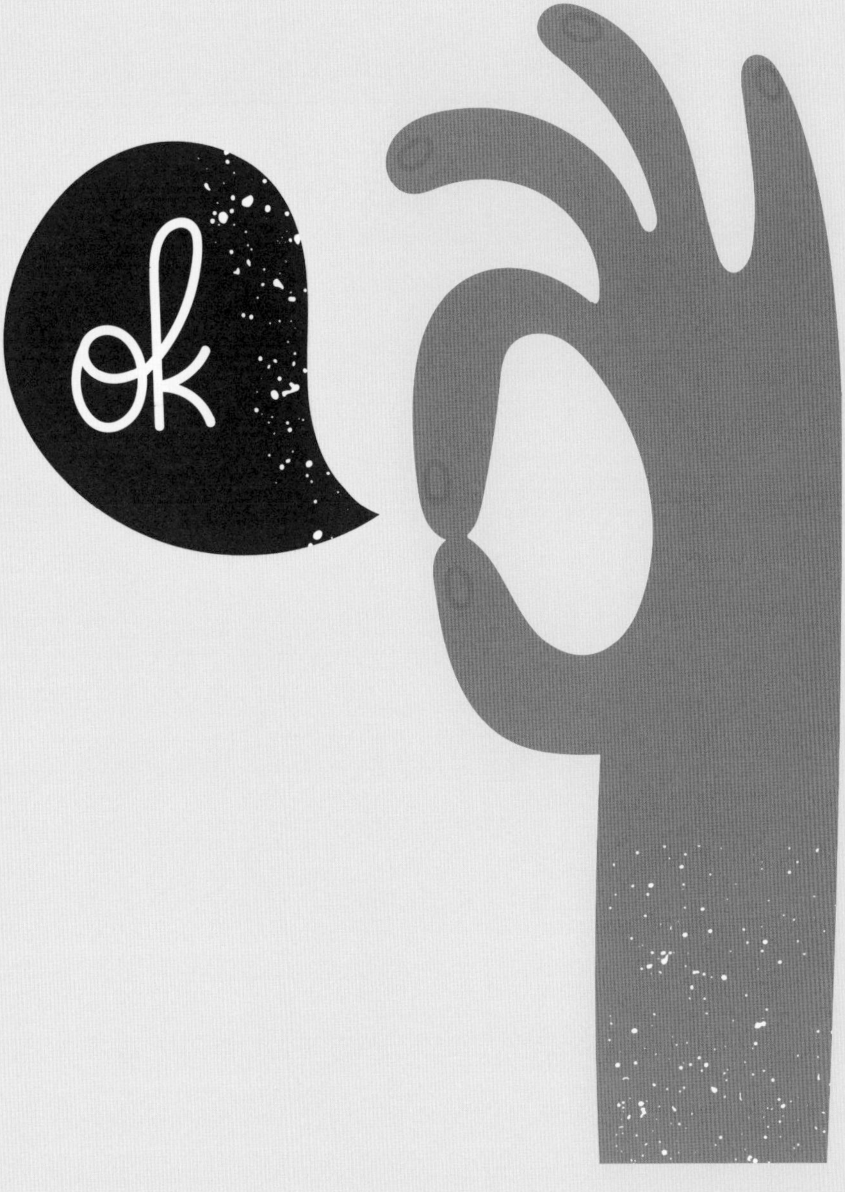
ok

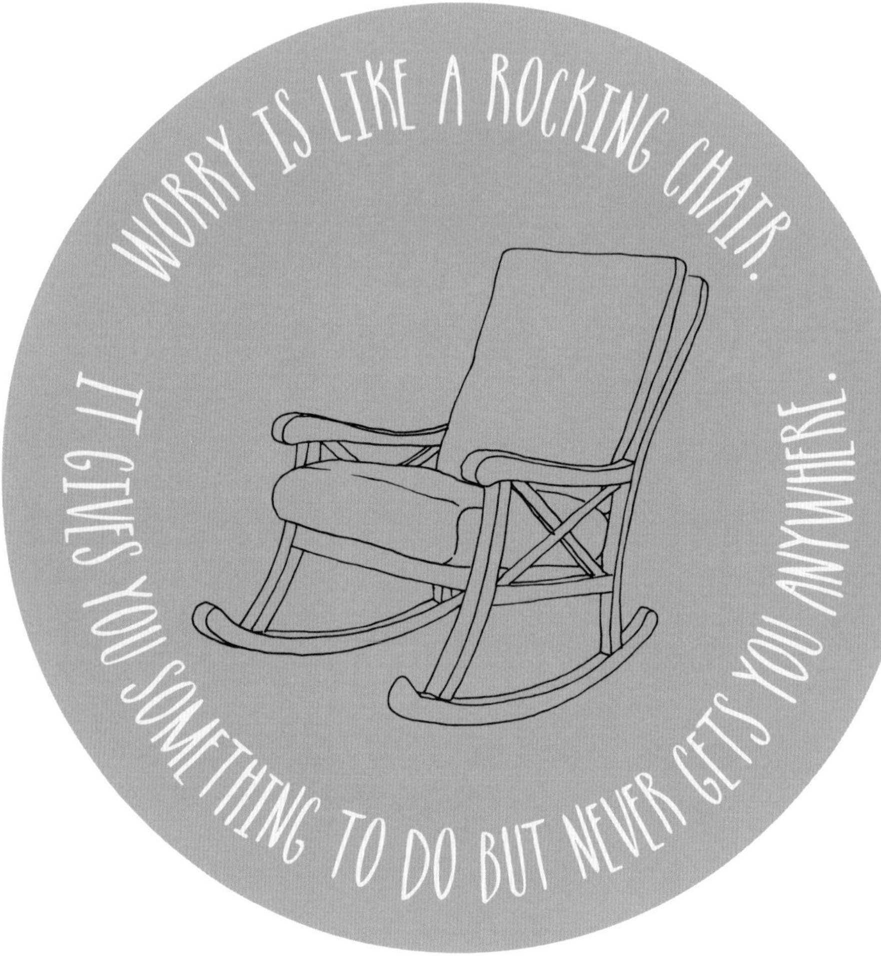

Erma Bombeck

Try mindful mantras

Find some positive phrases to keep you focused on your strengths. "I'm healthy and strong" might work for you if you want to get fitter, or "I believe in my own abilities" might be suitable if you are doubting yourself. Choose mantras you believe in and that resonate with you.

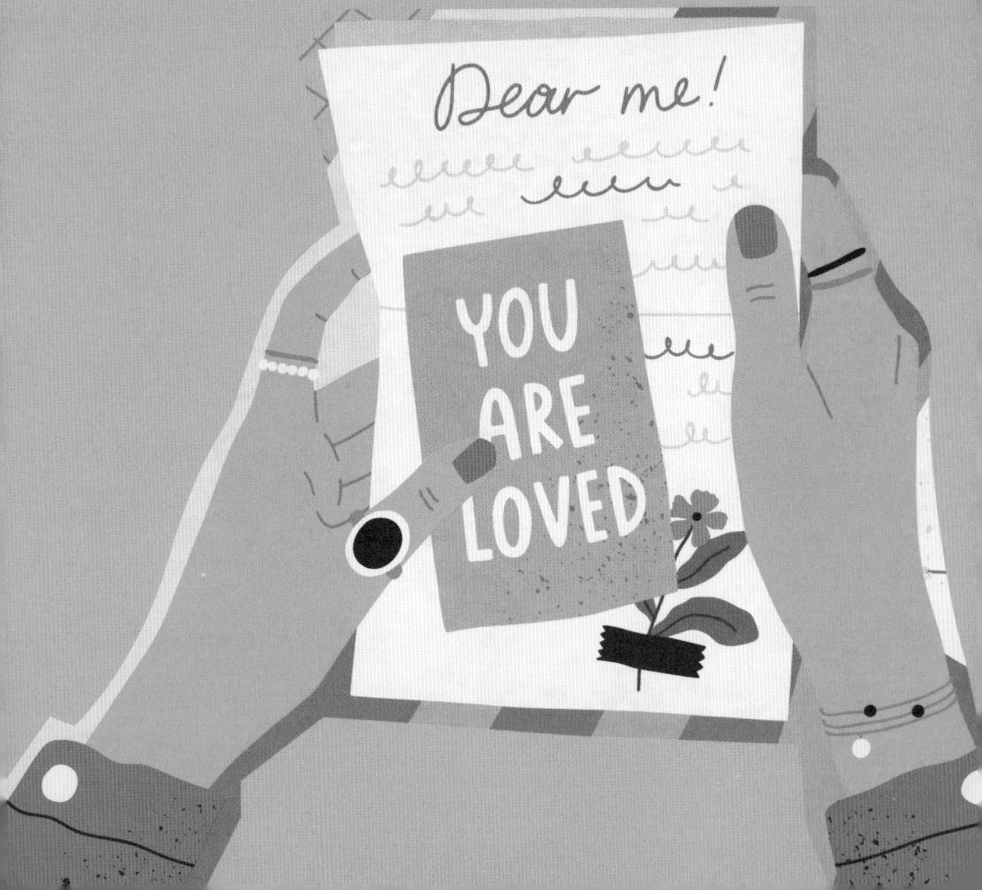

Help others

If you are prone to worrying too much, but feel you can't help it, try to shift the focus away from yourself onto something positive that involves helping others. Keep your mind busy so that you don't have time to overthink. For instance, if you are worried about an old friend not keeping in regular contact with you or not responding to your messages, you may worry you've done something to upset them. You might start to think all sorts of things, like "they think I'm no fun to be around" or "they find me boring". This may sound extreme, but when you don't have a purpose or a focus, it's easy to let negative thoughts fester. Try helping others less fortunate than you: volunteer at a charity shop or homeless centre and give a fresh purpose and focus to your overactive mind. This will stop you from sitting around wondering what might have gone wrong.

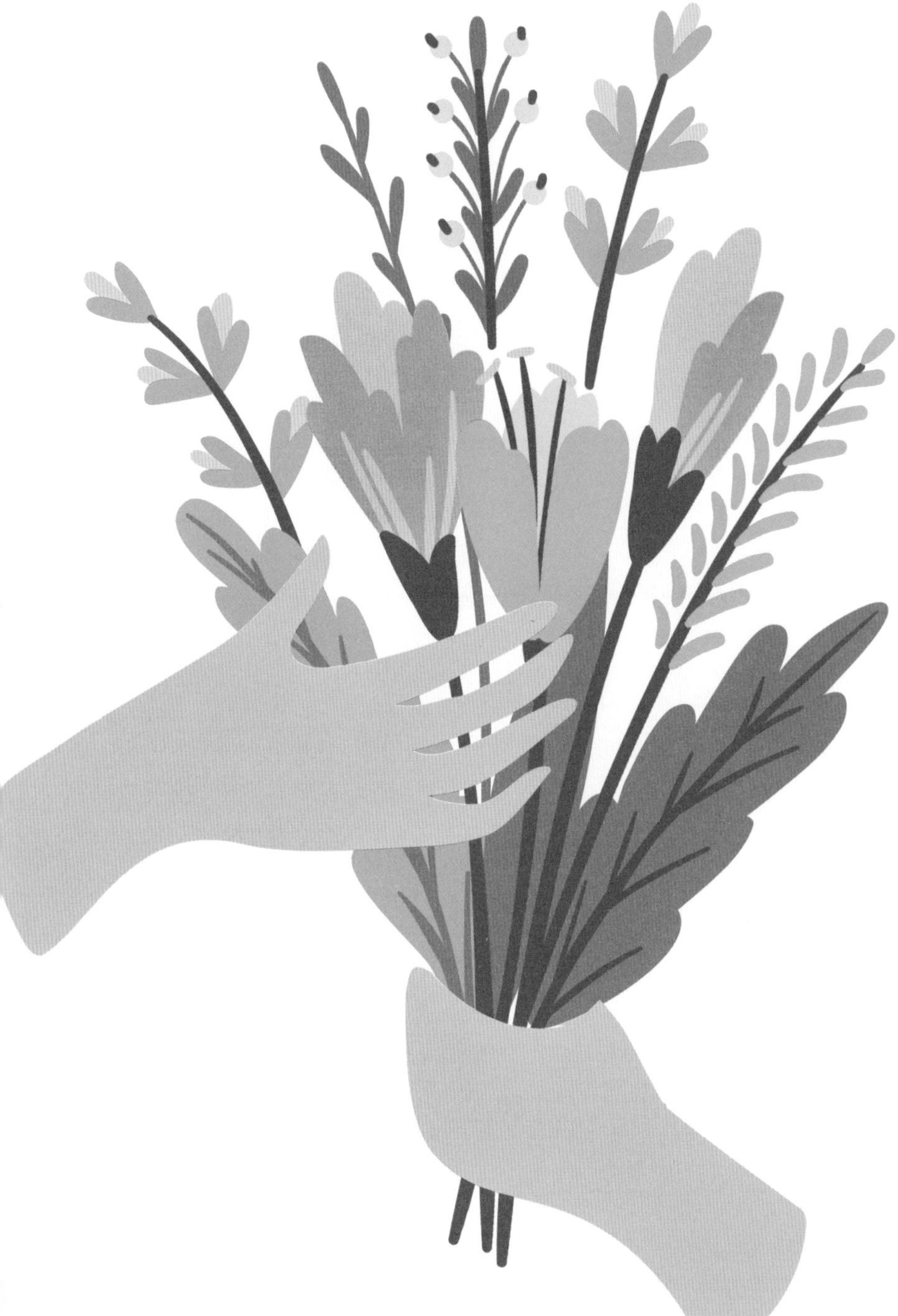

IF YOU DON'T GIVE UP, YOU STILL HAVE A CHANCE

Control your mindset

Anxiety is very much a state of mind... hopefully you can now see that thoughts can be controlled and managed and that they don't have to consume us entirely. How you respond to your thoughts is down to you. The next chapter looks at various ways to dispel your anxiety, from meditation to exercise and other mood-boosting ideas. There's much you can do to keep in control, so stay positive.

YOUR MIND IS A POWERFUL THING.
WHEN YOU FILL IT WITH POSITIVE THOUGHTS,
YOUR LIFE WILL START TO CHANGE.

John Assaraf

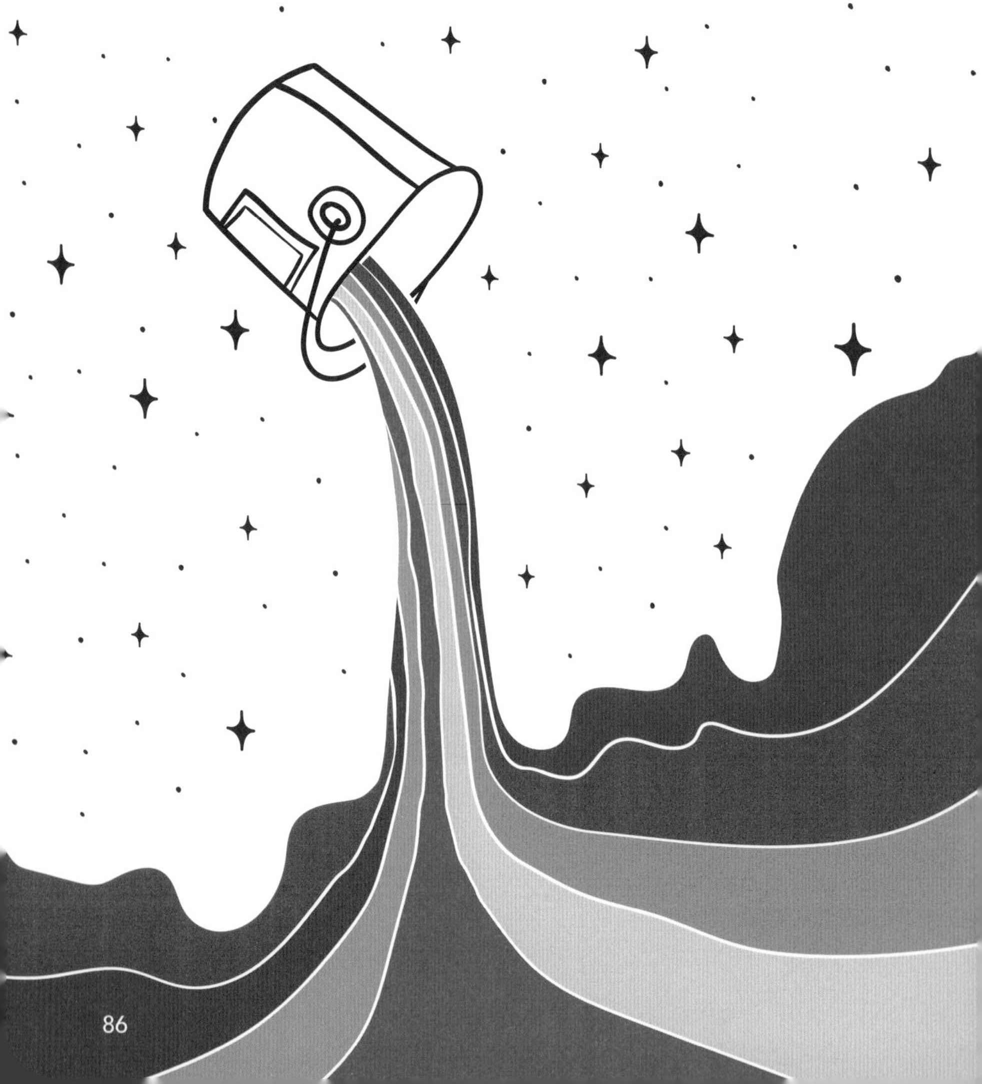

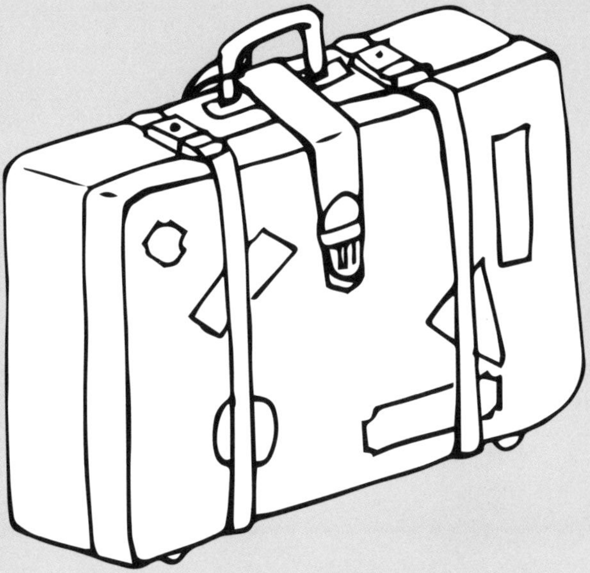

PART THREE:

SEND YOUR WORRIES PACKING

Whether your anxiety is caused by life being stressful or an overactive mind causing you to worry too much, there are various things you can do to restore calm and make you feel better. Even if you are dealing with a specific problem that can't be solved overnight, such as pressure at work or caring for a loved one, certain activities and pursuits will help you to develop the mental resilience to cope in the face of adversity.

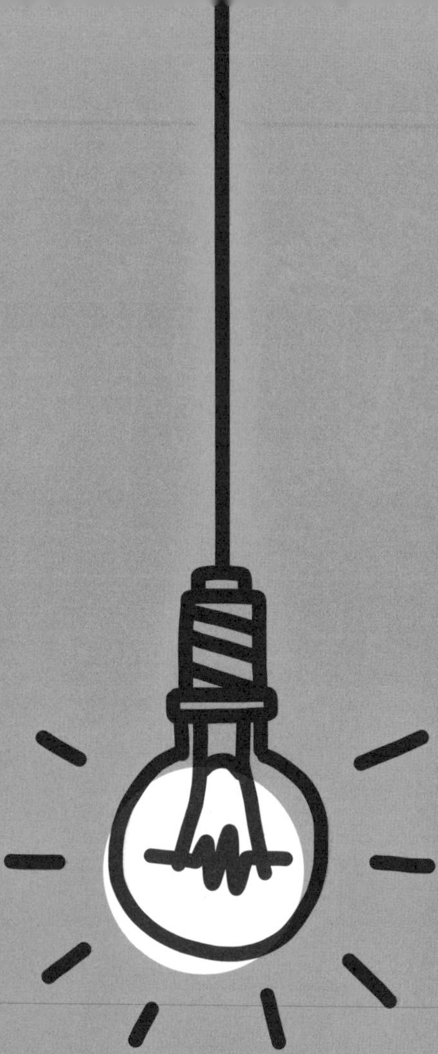

Appreciate the basics

If you're having a bad day, remind yourself of how fortunate you are to have friends and family, as well as the basics we often take for granted – such as food in the fridge, a roof over your head, clean water, electricity and heating. Sometimes, we undervalue these essential things and it can pay to remind ourselves to appreciate them.

Be thankful for the small things in life

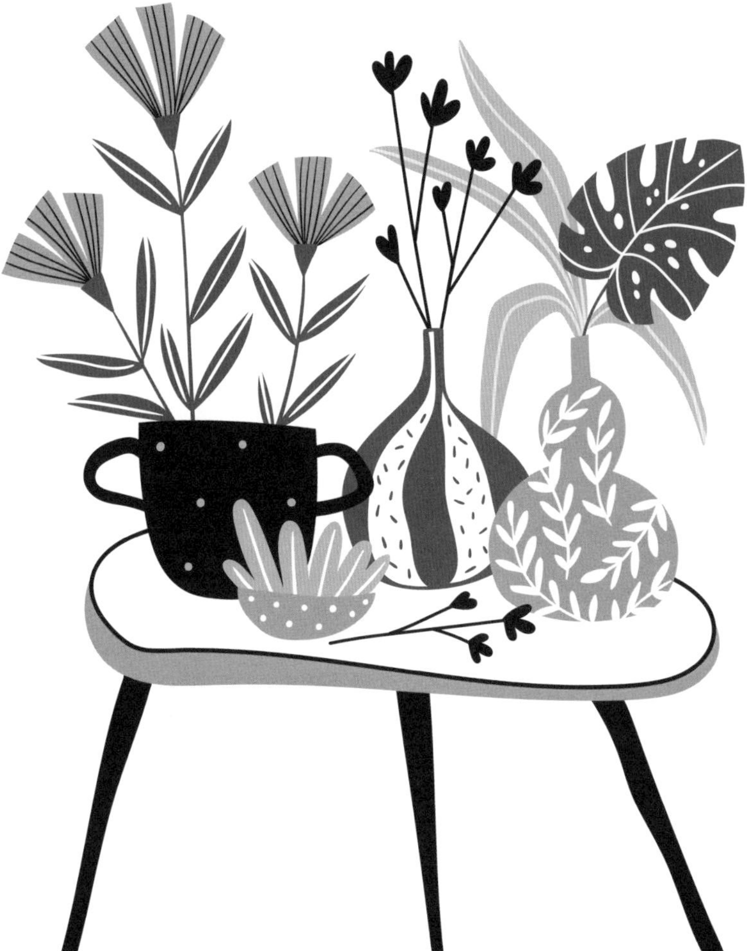

I think it's important to find the little things in everyday life that make you happy.

Paula Cole

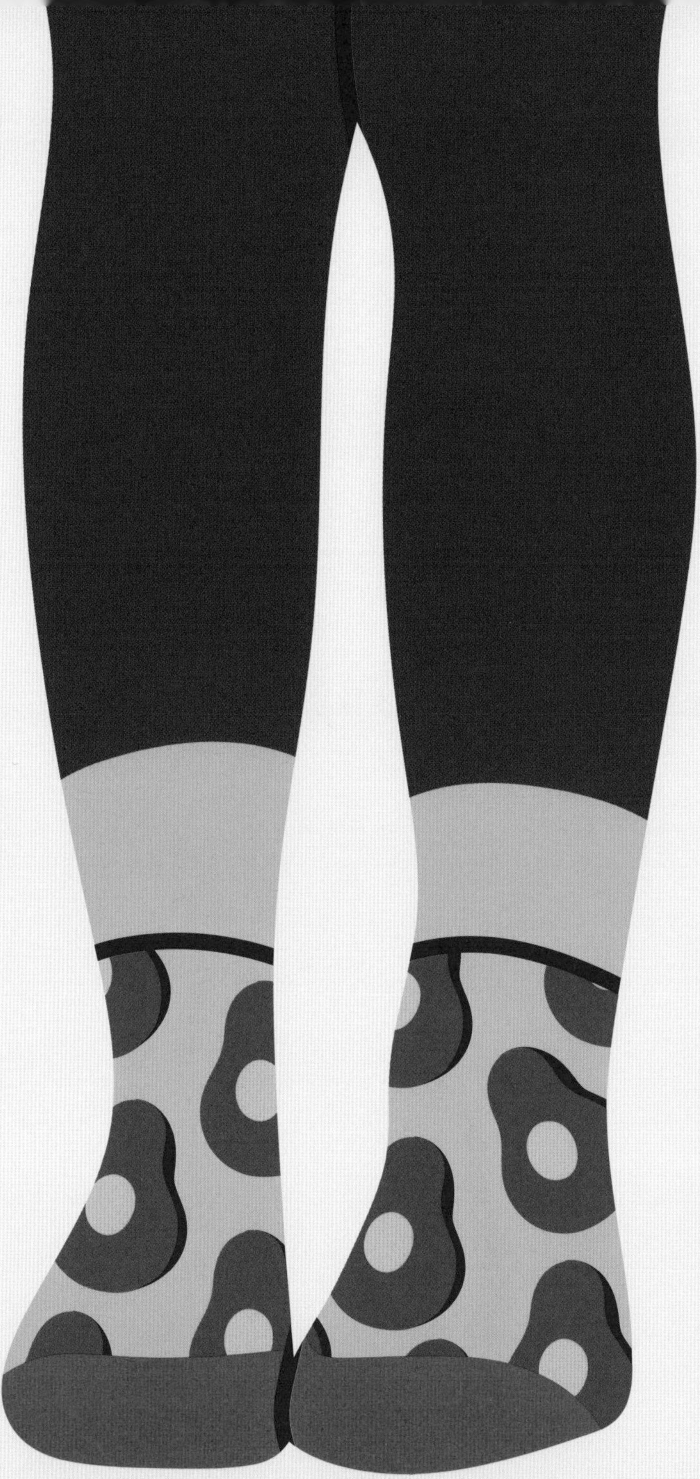

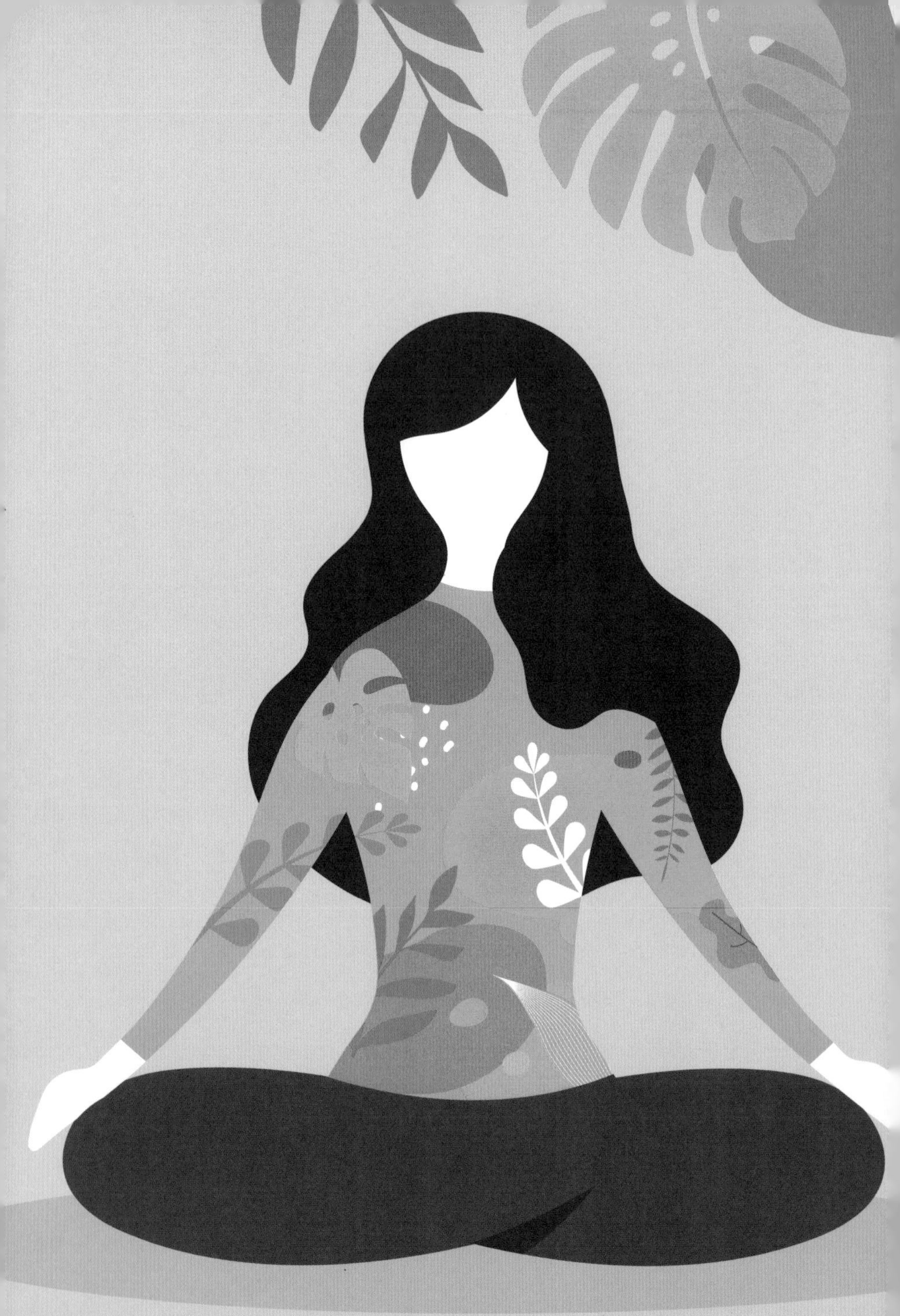

Practise mindfulness

If you are anxious and find yourself worrying a lot of the time, mindfulness can be very effective at calming your mind. You don't need any equipment – just a quiet space at home or at work in your lunch break. Mindfulness is about being reflective rather than reactive to what's going on around you and focusing on the present moment, rather than on the future. Mindfulness can help to reduce anxiety and depression and has been recognized internationally for its mental health benefits. It encourages us to accept our emotions, become more aware of our bodies, focus our attention and be more conscious of ourselves. To practise mindfulness, focus on your breathing and feel your chest rise and fall. Concentrate on what's going on in the present moment; the sights and sounds around you. If you find your mind wandering onto things you've got to do later that day, that's OK – just bring it back to the present moment. Employ mindfulness whenever you feel stressed.

Count your blessings with gratitude

SET PEACE OF MIND AS YOUR HIGHEST GOAL AND ORGANIZE YOUR LIFE AROUND IT.

Brian Tracy

Inhale courage, exhale fear

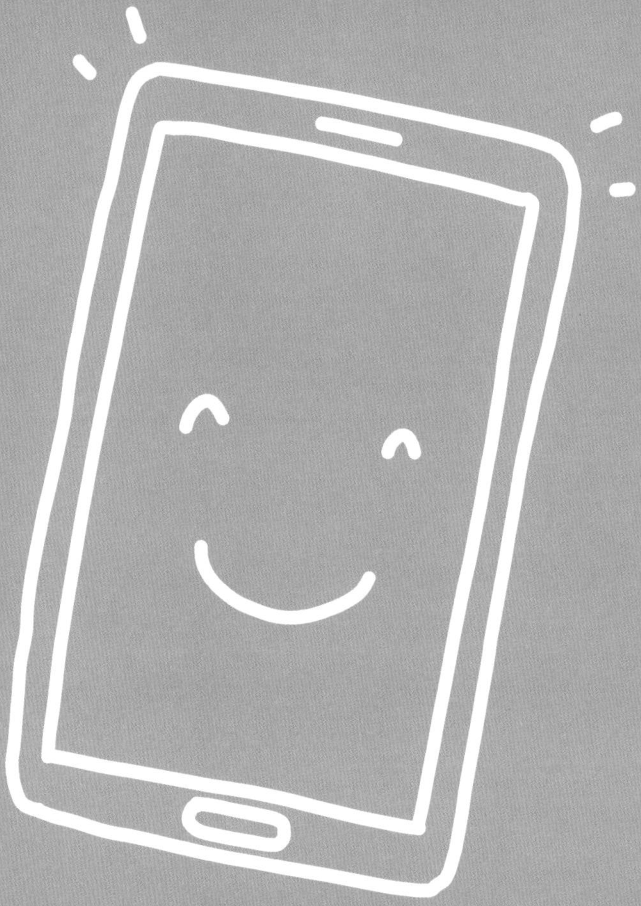

Unfollow negativity

Though social media can be fun, it can sometimes feel like a platform for negativity to spread. It can be easy to get pulled into a stream of disheartening comments being shared and posted about politics, climate change or the world we live in today. Unfollow anyone who has a habit of posting negative comments and stick with the humorous or upbeat posts. Funny pet videos are always a win–win!

A RUFFLED MIND MAKES

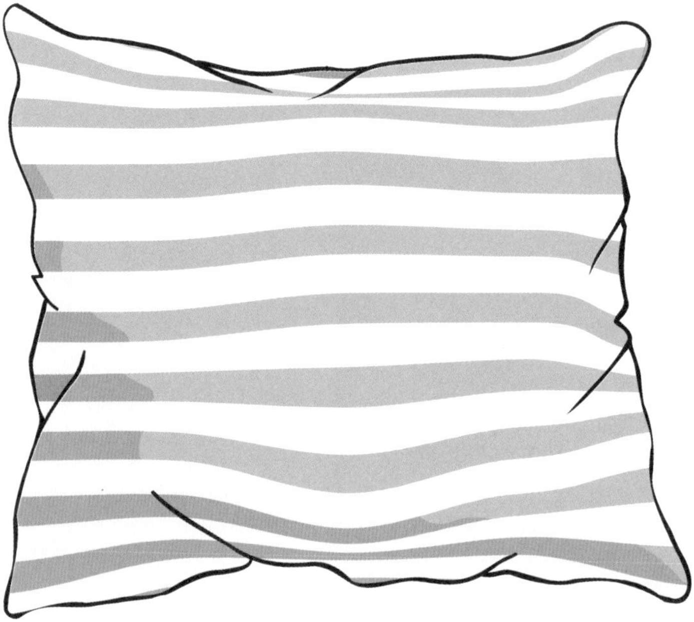

A RESTLESS PILLOW.

Charlotte Brontë

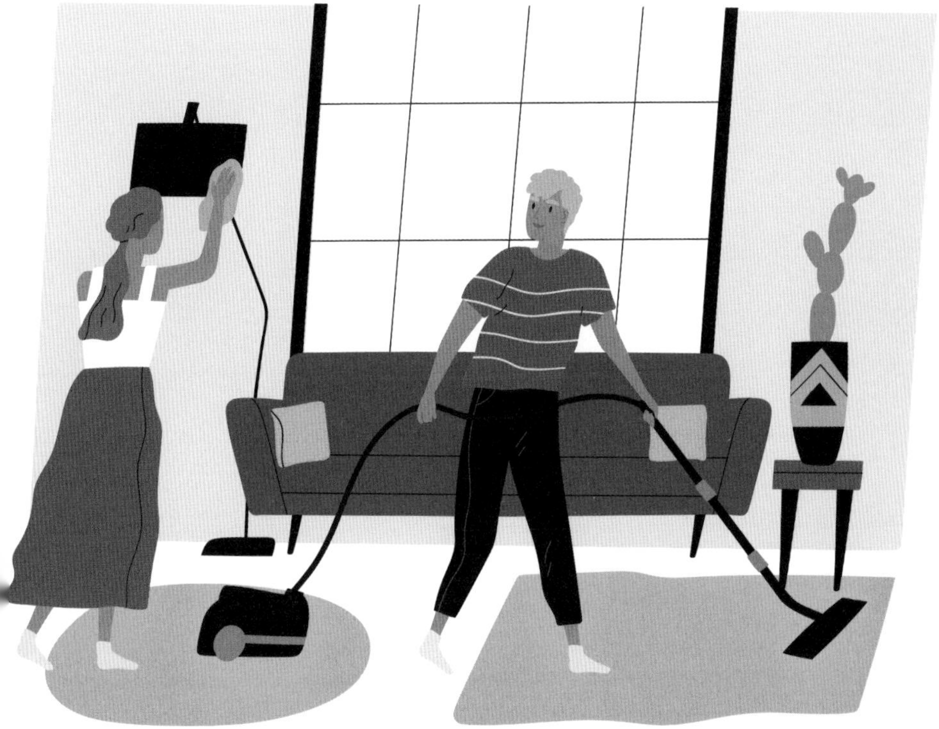

Clear the clutter

Reduce anxiety by clearing some clutter around the house and tidying up. It doesn't have to be an all-out spring clean – perhaps just sort out a messy drawer or organize your desk or kitchen worktop. Completing small tasks like this won't overwhelm you and will make you feel that you have accomplished a worthwhile task. What's more, an uncluttered space can help you to think more clearly. A tidy home equals a tidy mind!

Embrace health and fitness

Health is one of the most precious commodities we have, yet we often don't fully appreciate it until we become ill. As the saying goes, "those who don't find time for health will sooner or later have to find time for illness". Regular cardiovascular exercise like cycling, running, jogging, brisk walking or exercise classes that raise your heart rate are all beneficial for heart health and reducing your risk of diseases like cancer and dementia. However, having a life that just involves work, exercise and no down-time will not be good for you in the long term either. Try to adopt a good balance in your life.

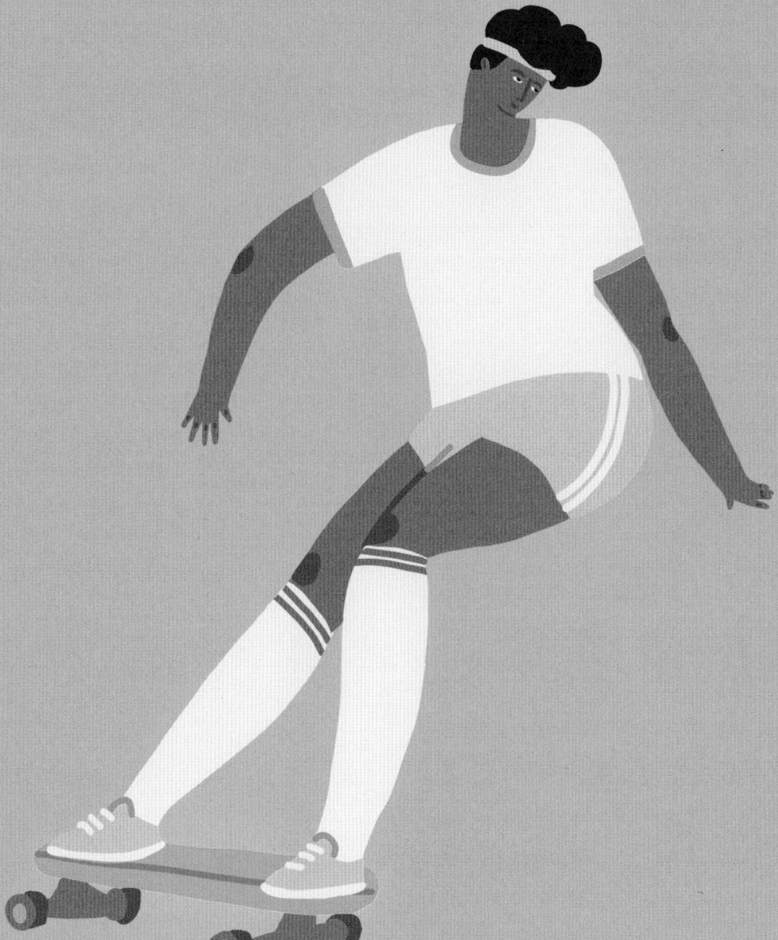

Accept what you can't control

There are some things you can't control, like other people's moods and behaviour and how they talk about you, or what has happened in the past. Let go of negativity and stop trying to influence the opinions, actions and behaviour of others; let them be responsible for themselves. The minute you start to put yourself first, you'll begin to feel better.

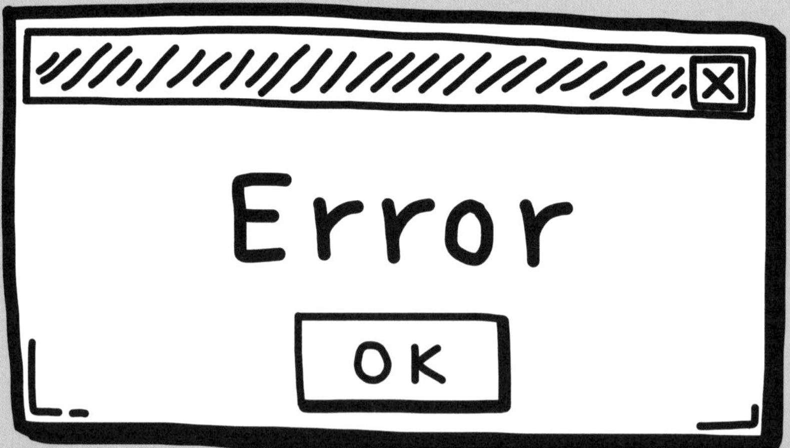

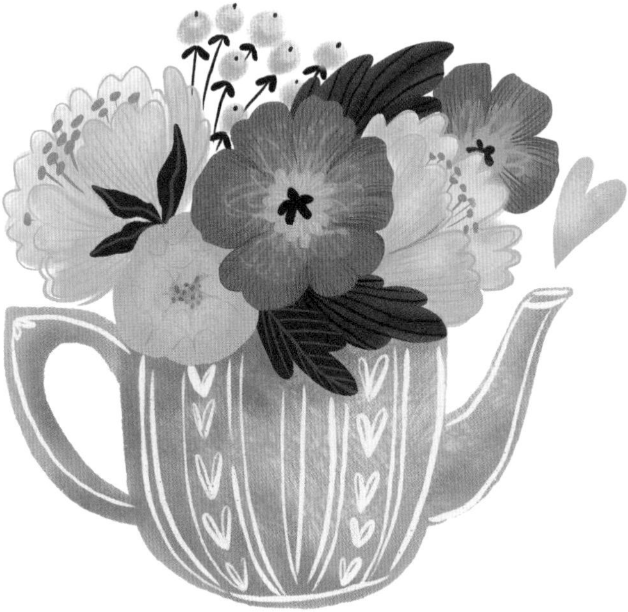

Beautiful things happen when you distance yourself from negativity

Of all the liars in the world,

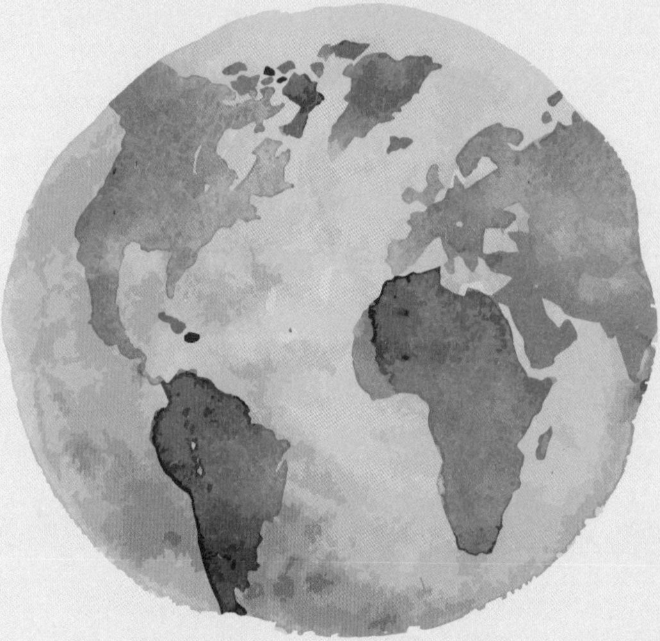

sometimes the worst are our own fears.

Rudyard Kipling

Will it matter in five years?

If you are worried about a specific problem, ask yourself if it will matter in five years' time. If it won't matter in five years, then don't spend more than five minutes worrying about it. You can apply this whenever something happens to cause you upset. Sometimes you might say "yes, it will matter", but asking yourself the question will help you understand that what you are worried about is important and requires deep thought. Otherwise, let it go.

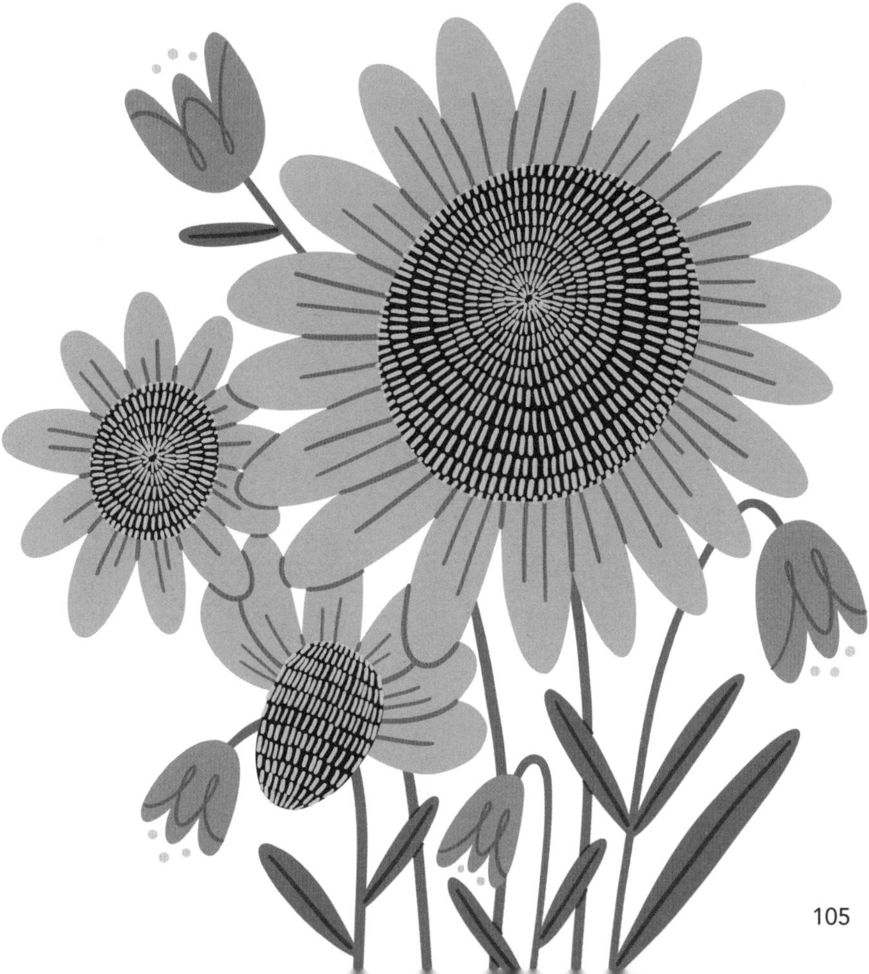

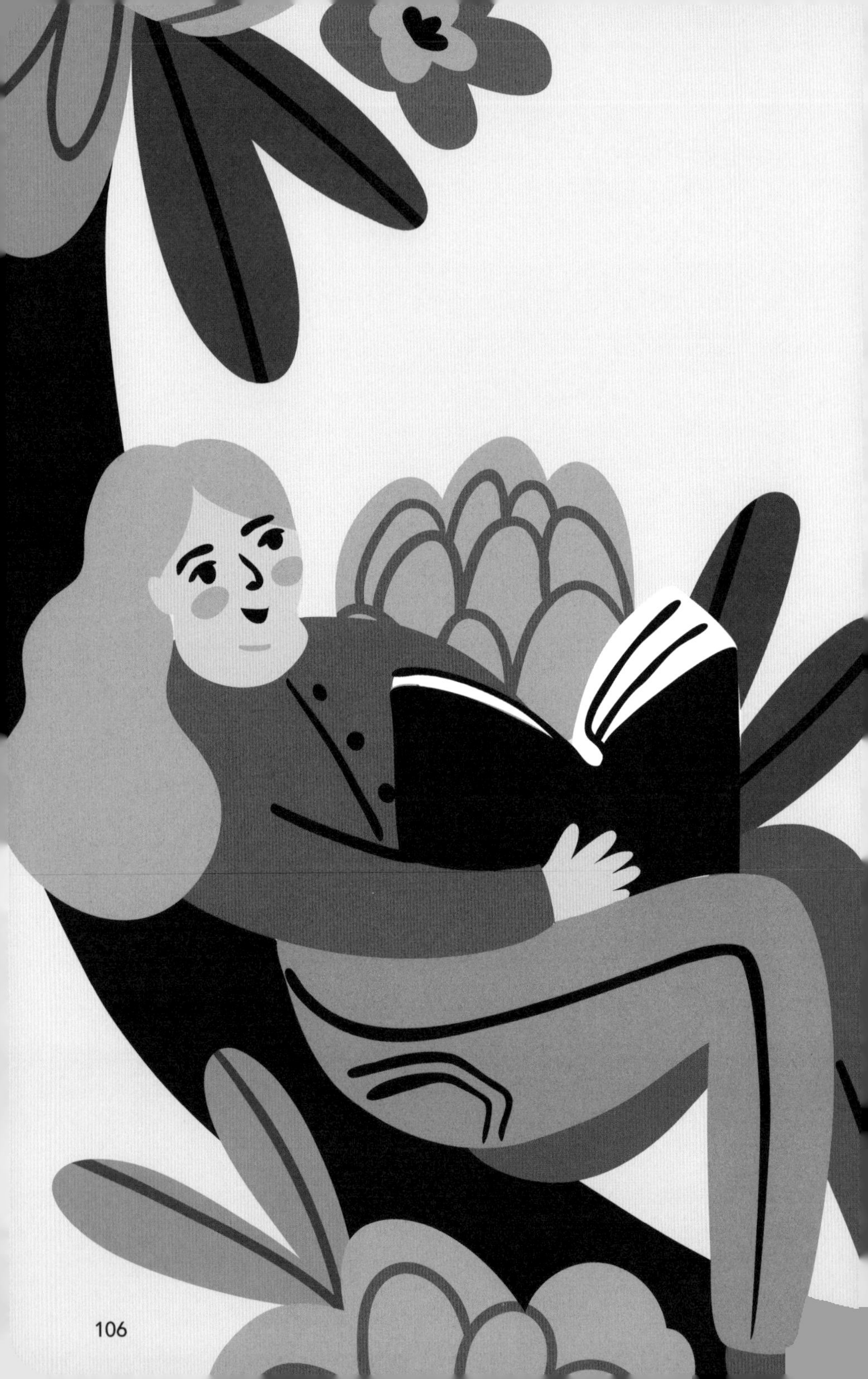

Create the life you want

Worry and frustration can come from feeling that your life is out of your control. If you feel you're not leading the life you want, think about the future you'd like to create for yourself and work out how you can reach it. Visualize what your new life would be like and write down your goals. Imagine how incredible it will feel to achieve new objectives or to make the changes you want to make. Then think about how good it will feel to be in control of your own destiny. Start to implement changes that will move you closer to your goal – whatever it may be – so that you feel you are taking positive steps toward creating your ideal future. Plan and prepare now. Even if you just make small, gradual changes, it's worth getting started; it will give you renewed energy and a positive focus.

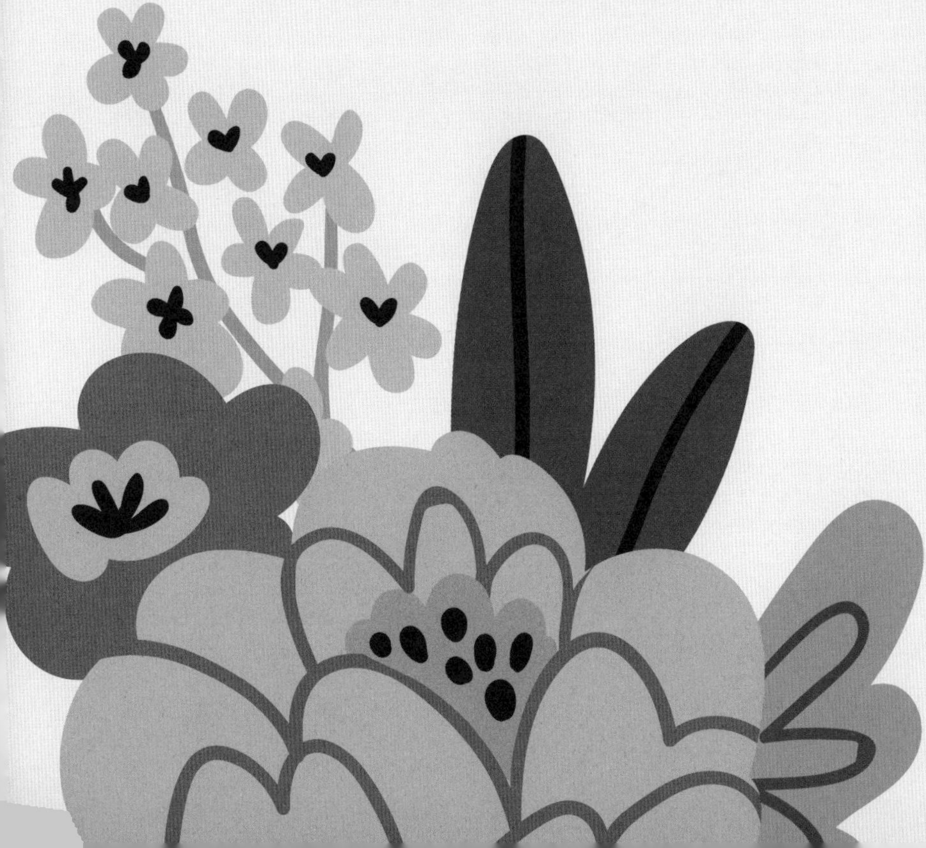

The day you stop worrying will be the first day of

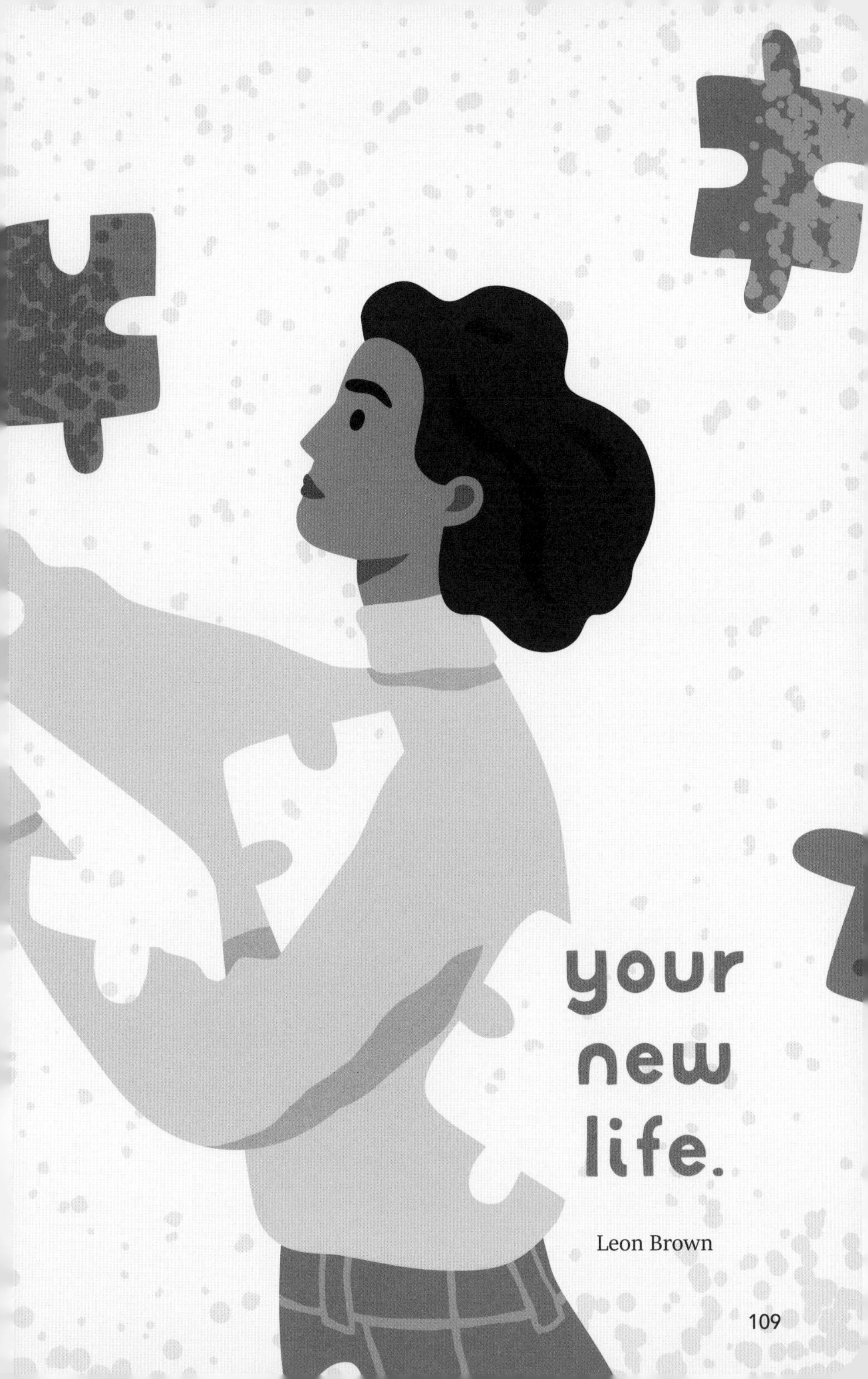
your
new
life.
Leon Brown

Make yourself a priority

Many of us find it hard to say no when it comes to helping others or accommodating their wishes in some way. Work on being more assertive and putting your needs first. If you spend all of your time trying to please other people, you may begin to feel worn out, put upon and taken for granted. Make sure you put yourself first when you need to. It's not a selfish act – it's necessary. The following saying is true: "You can't pour from an empty cup."

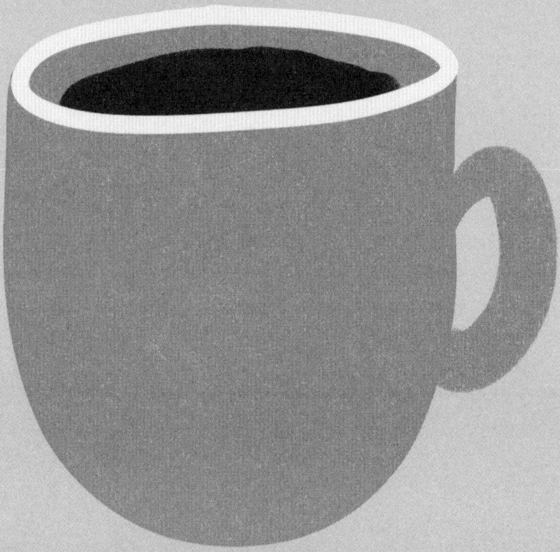

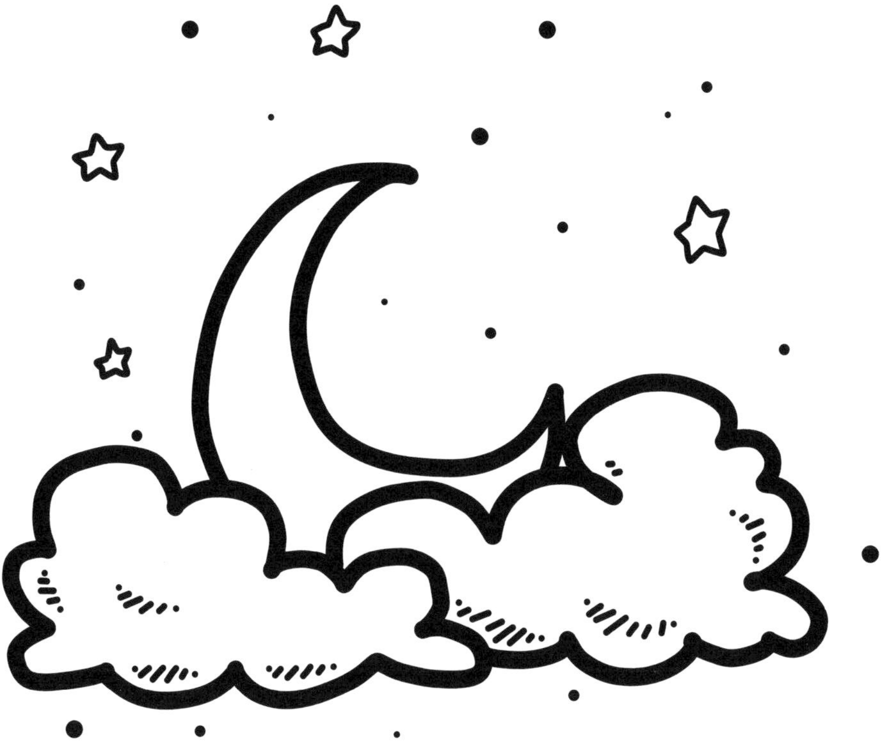

REMEMBER,
TODAY IS THE
TOMORROW YOU
WORRIED ABOUT
YESTERDAY.

Dale Carnegie

Take an active break

Next time you feel anxious, get moving. Exercise decreases hormones like cortisol, which is responsible for our "fight or flight" response and is produced when our body is exposed to prolonged stress or anxiety. It also releases endorphins – these are chemicals produced by the nervous system to help us cope with stress and act as a pain reliever. If you're worrying about something, while exercise in itself won't solve the issue, it will reduce your stress levels and improve your ability to cope with stressful situations. A quick run, a brisk walk or simply doing some stretching on a mat at home will almost certainly make you feel better.

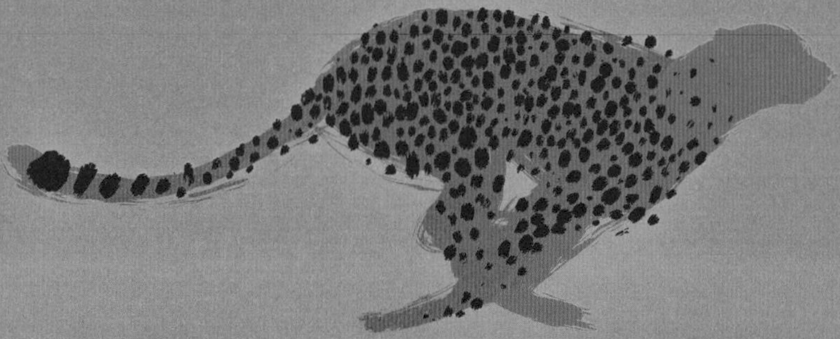

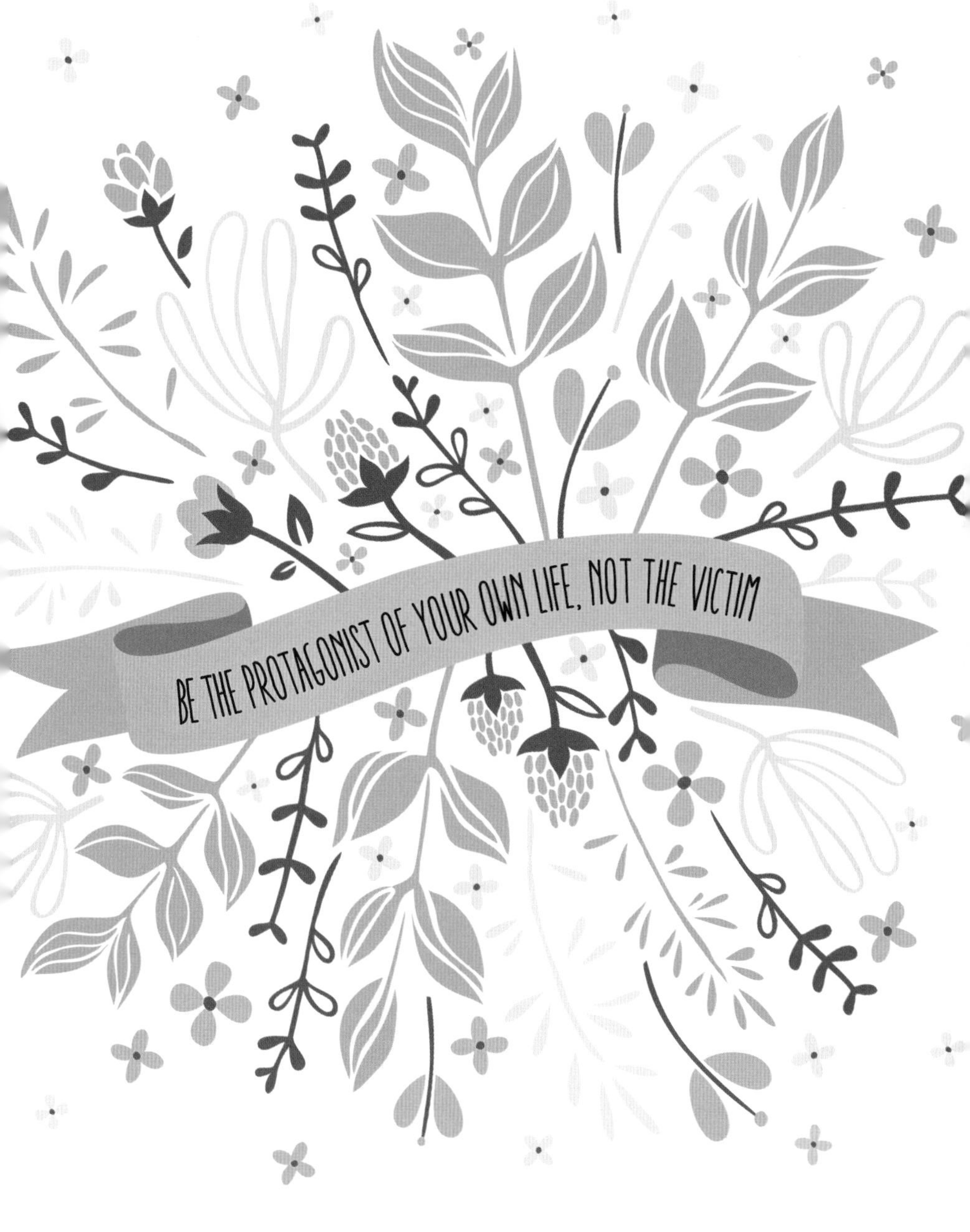
BE THE PROTAGONIST OF YOUR OWN LIFE, NOT THE VICTIM

Give yoga a go

The mental health benefits of yoga are well known, so it could be the solution to help you feel calmer and less stressed. Yoga helps to relieve physical discomfort through various yoga poses – or "asanas" – which help to stretch, lengthen and balance your muscles and reduce muscle tension and inflammation. If your body is more relaxed and you don't have any aches, you are more likely to feel happier and enjoy a sense of calm and ease. Practising yoga has also been shown to increase the level of a brain chemical called gamma-aminobutyric acid (GABA), which helps to regulate nerve activity. Its benefits are backed up by research, too. A 2018 study, published in the peer-reviewed journal *Complementary Therapies in Clinical Practice*, found that yoga can lower your heart rate and blood pressure, reduce your stress response, depression and anxiety, and increase feelings of energy and well-being.

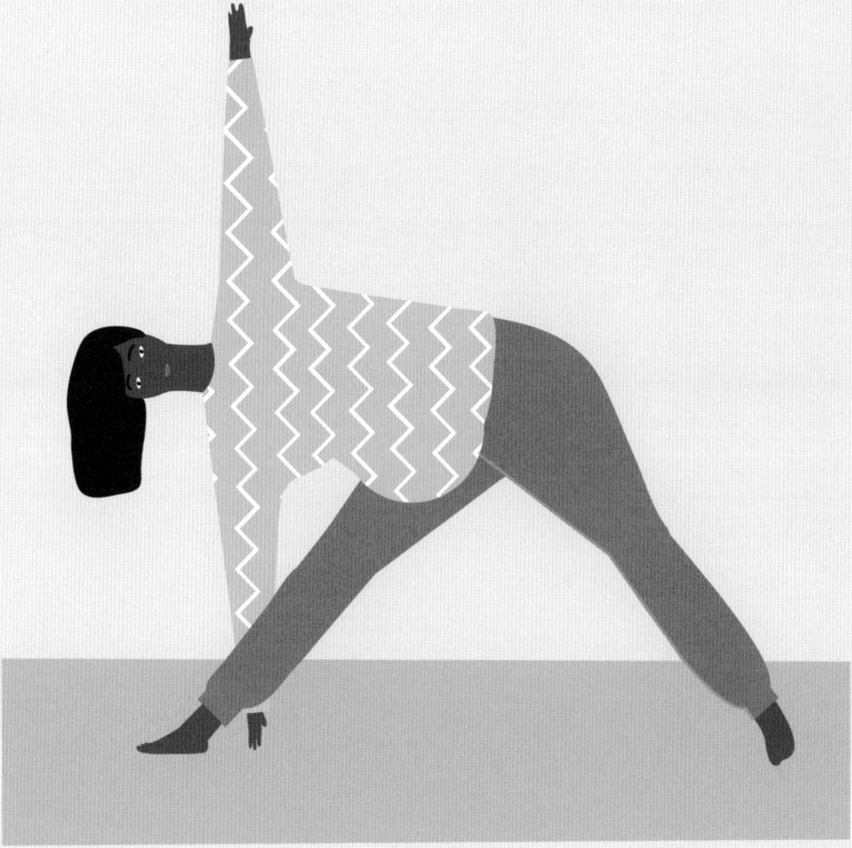

Inner peace begins the moment you choose not to allow another person or event to control your emotions.

Pema Chodron

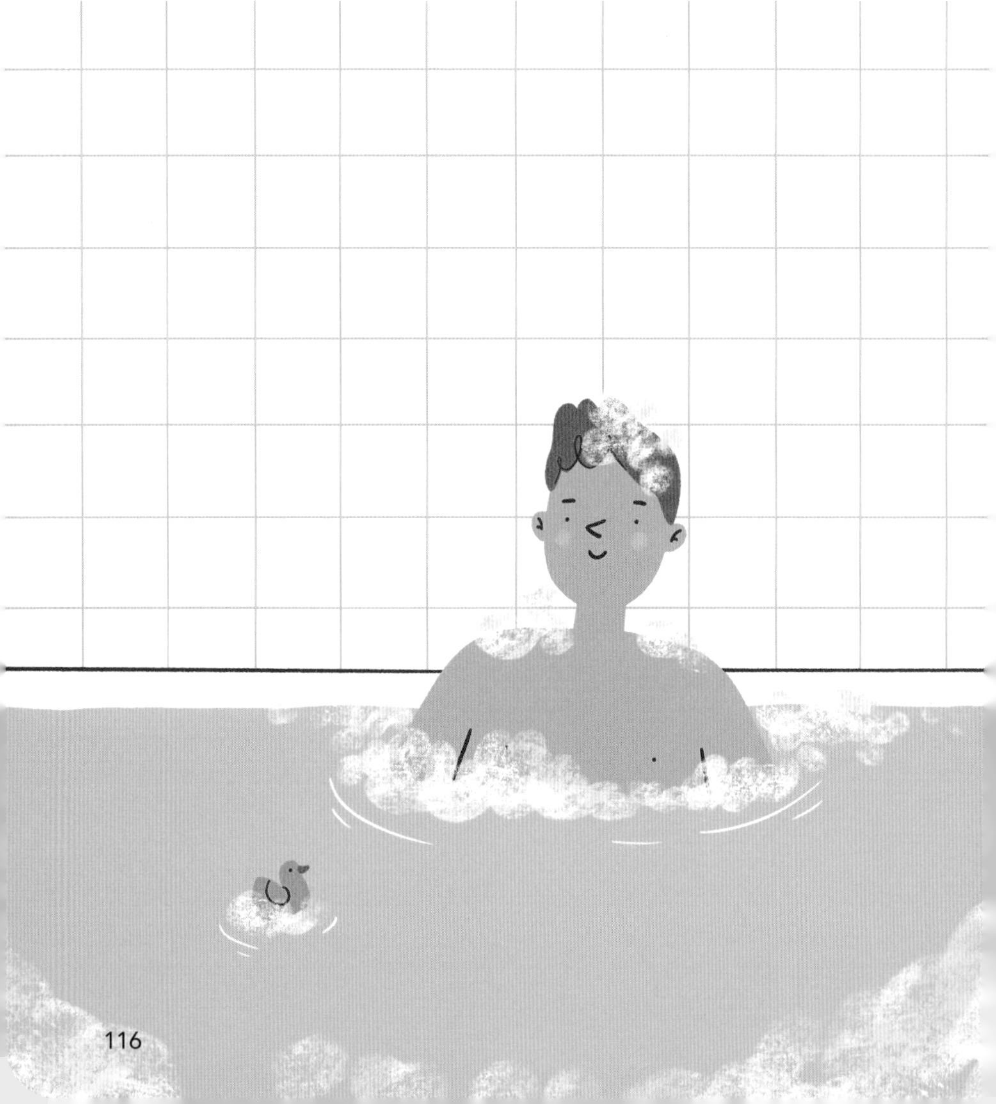

Get outside

Exercise outdoors when you can. According to the charity Mind, the sights, sounds and smells of nature – especially in green spaces – can have a calming effect on the mind and boost your mental health. It doesn't have to be strenuous exercise either; going for a walk in your local park or around a field will do the trick.

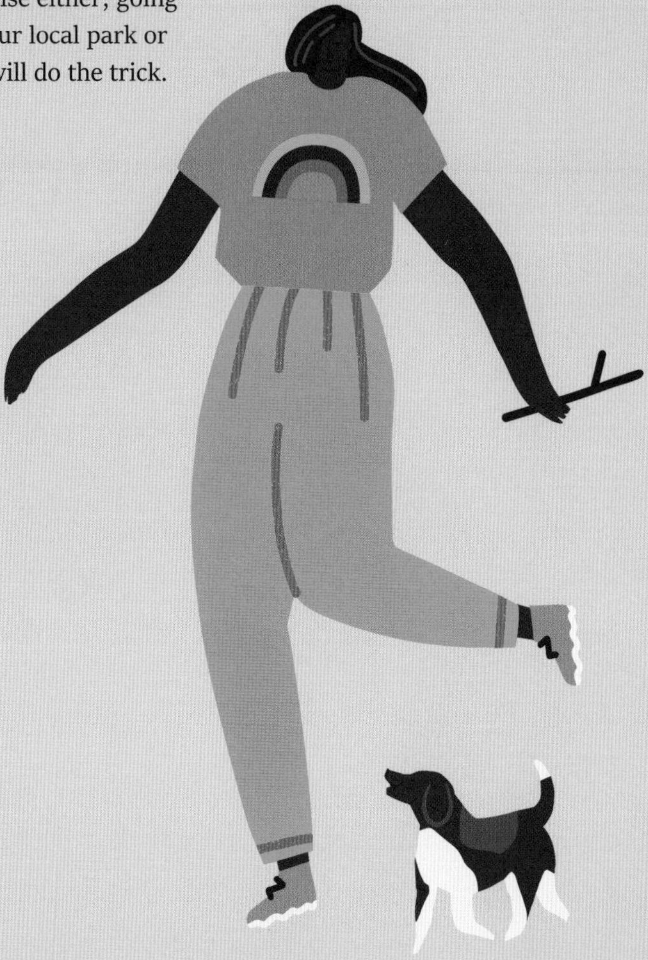

Be more cat

For a calmer outlook, live your life like a cat. Felines instinctively know what they need – they nap when they need to, eat when they are hungry and do what they want, without worrying about others. If that sounds a bit too ruthless, then try to take on some of their traits – or simply enjoy the company of a pet. A study presented at a US conference in 2008 showed that owning a cat can reduce your risk of heart attack and stroke by more than a third; even just stroking a cat had the potential to lower blood pressure.

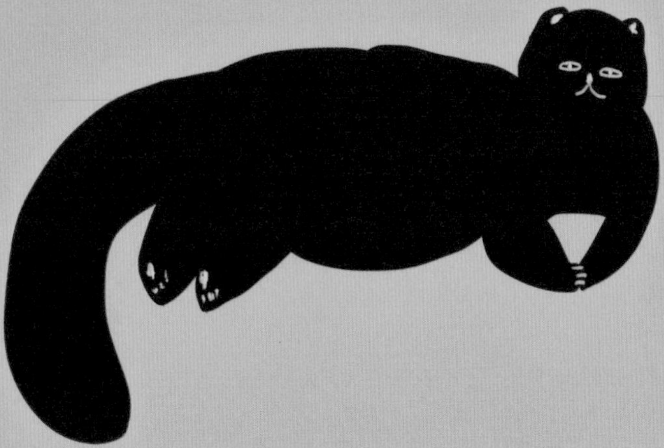

LIFE IS ONLY AS GOOD AS YOUR MINDSET

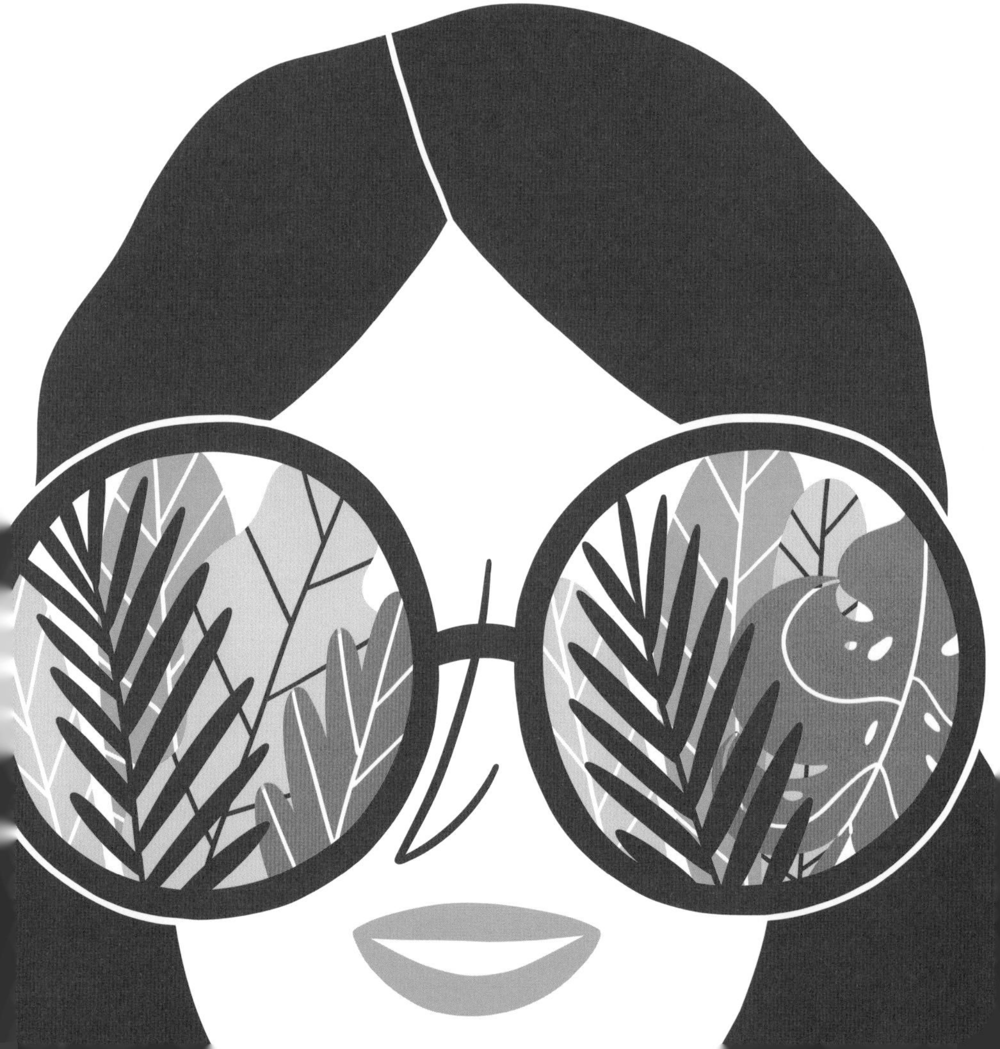

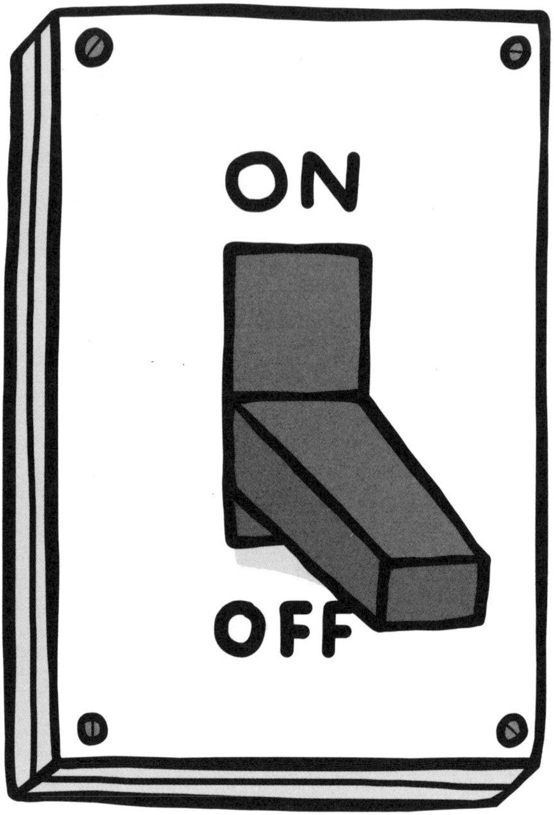

THE GREATEST WEAPON AGAINST STRESS IS OUR ABILITY TO CHOOSE ONE THOUGHT OVER ANOTHER.

William James

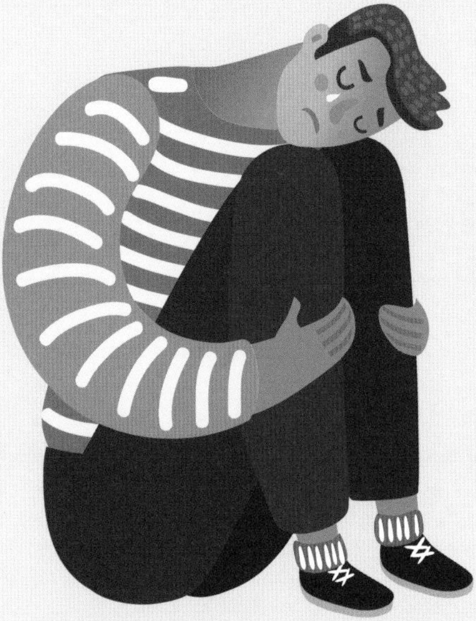

Be patient with bereavements

If you have recently lost a loved one, such as a parent, elderly relative or even worse, a close partner, you will be dealing with all sorts of mixed emotions – and anxiousness can be one of them. It's important to deal with bereavements after a loved one has died, as there is a tendency to develop an awareness of your own mortality and become fearful. Speak to someone who can help. Be patient with yourself. It can take up to several years or more to fully come to terms with the loss.

ATTITUDE IS EVERYTHING

PART FOUR:

LIVING WITH ANXIETY

We can try to deal with anxiety by managing our emotions and questioning negative thoughts when they come into our head. Sometimes though, while you can do your best to combat negativity, it's also important to realize that it's OK to not be OK. There is nothing to be ashamed of in seeking help – either from friends, family or from a health professional. Talking your worries through with a third party will make you feel better.

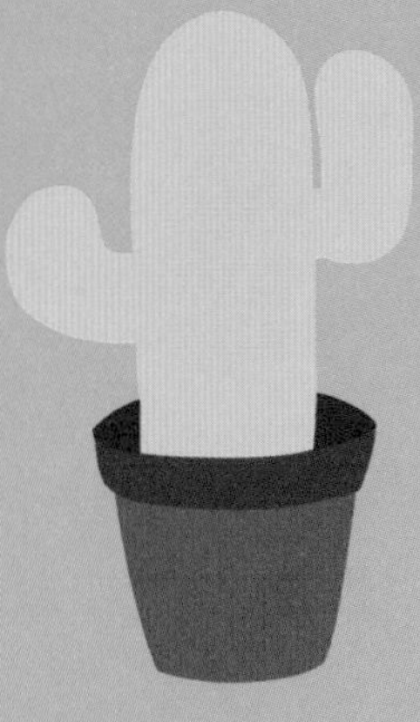

Have “worry windows”

Try to distinguish between thinking and worrying. Thinking is constructive and can help you to solve problems and improve situations. Worrying needlessly can cause catastrophizing, where you imagine the worst-case scenario and work yourself up into a stressed state. Rather than constantly worrying, and therefore making it a habit you are unconsciously developing, have “worry periods”. Allocate a pre-determined amount of time to deal with issues that are bothering you and hopefully generate possible solutions or ways of managing your stress.

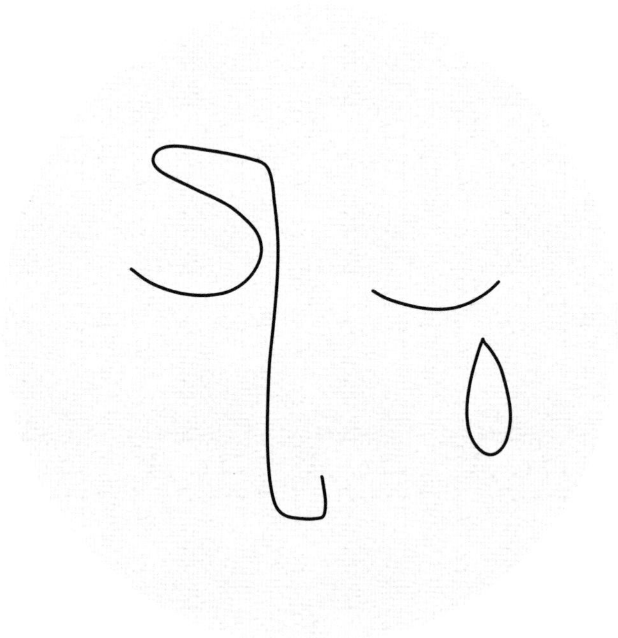

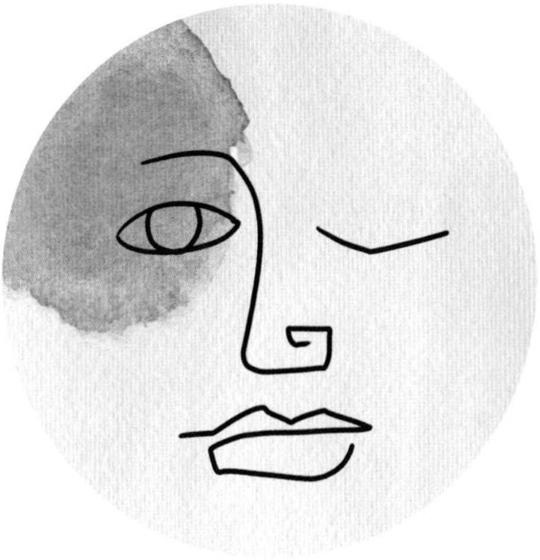

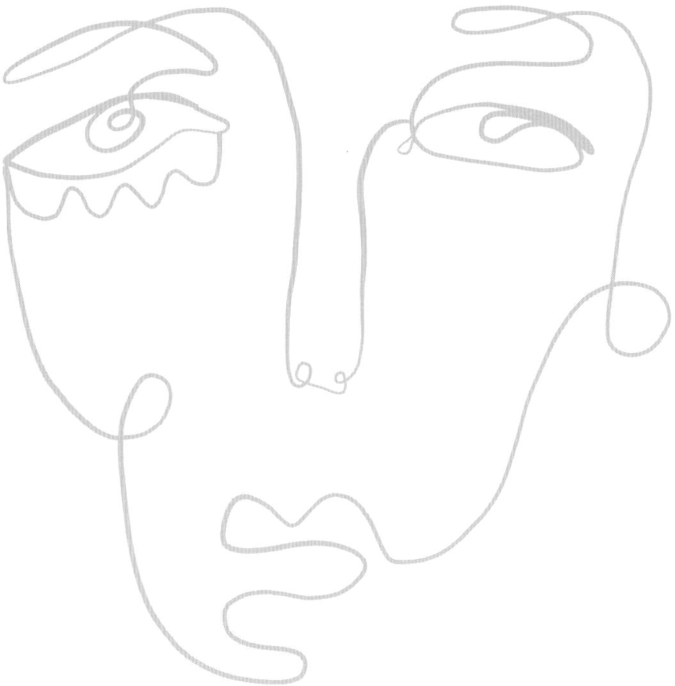

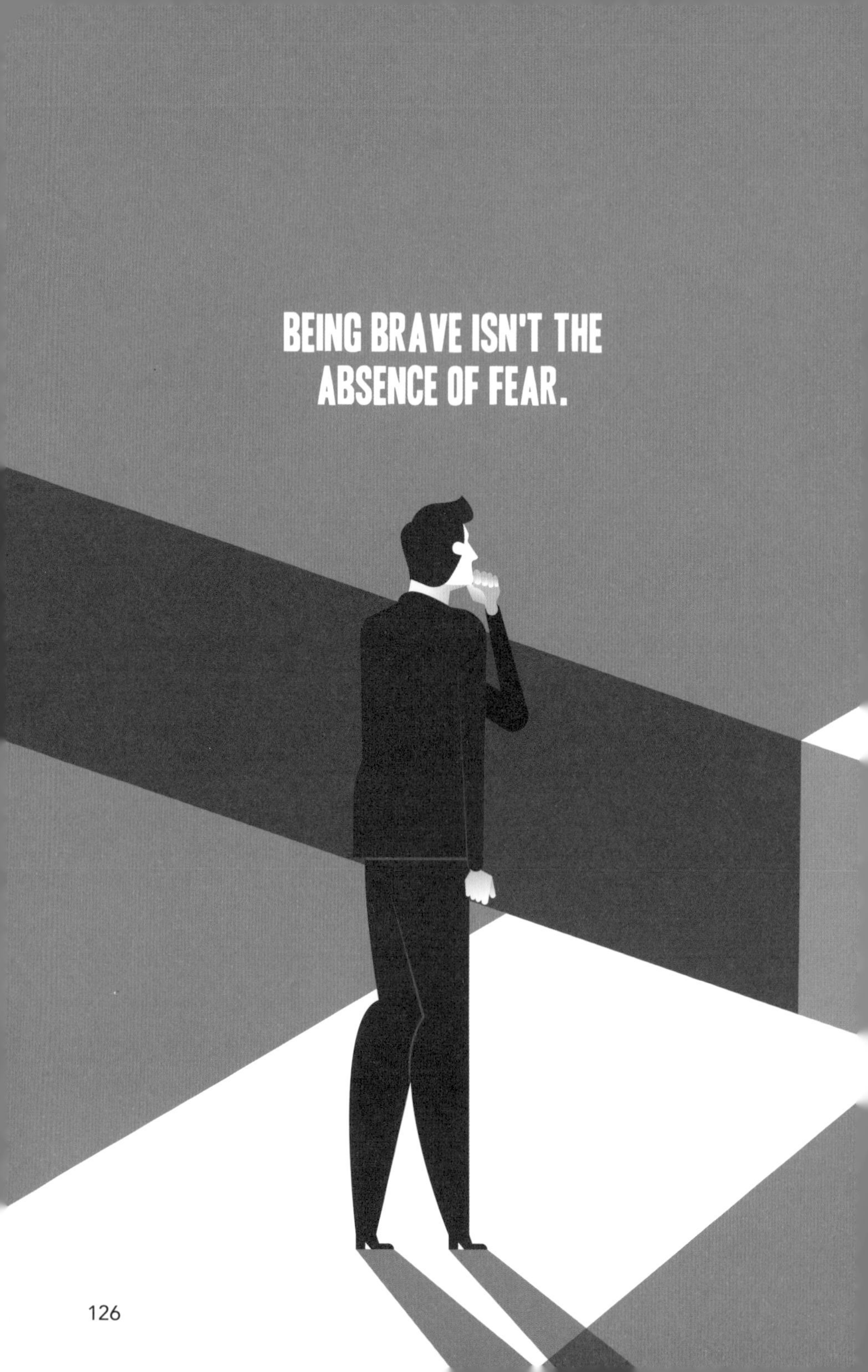
BEING BRAVE ISN'T THE
ABSENCE OF FEAR.

BEING BRAVE IS HAVING THAT FEAR BUT FINDING A WAY THROUGH IT.

Bear Grylls

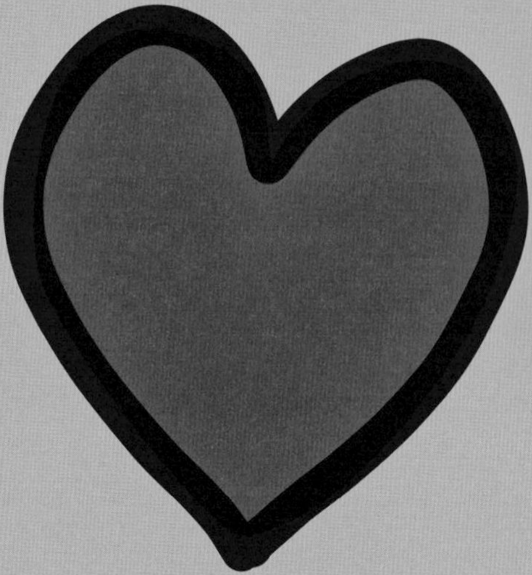

Anxiety weighs down the heart, but a kind word cheers it up

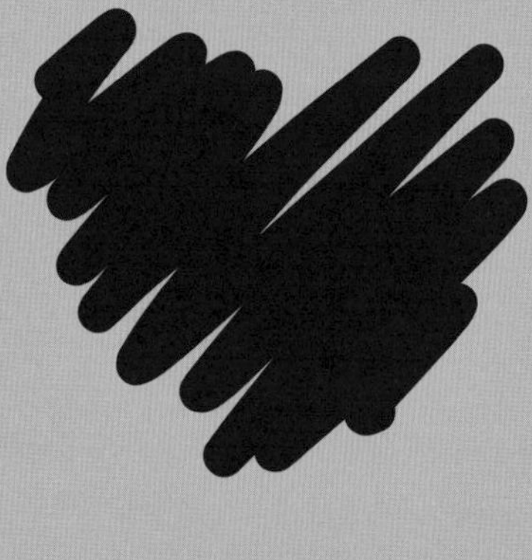

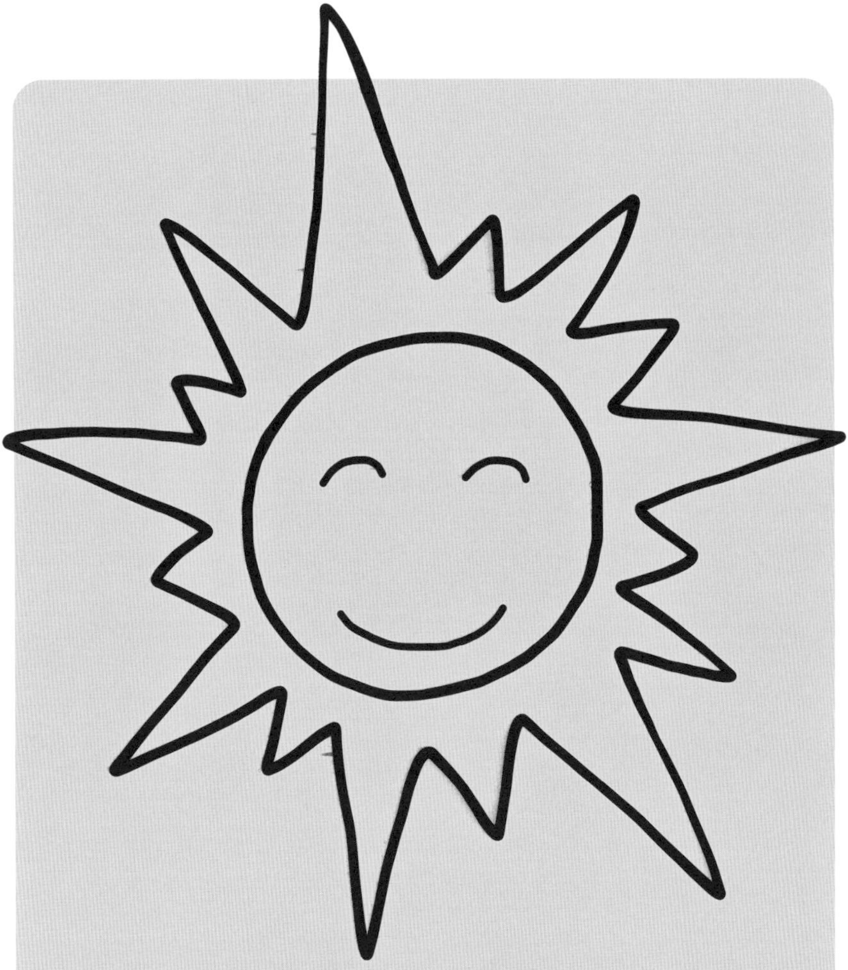

Share a positive outlook

Get into a habit of positive thinking. It may feel more natural on some days than others, but try to be someone who sees the up-side in every situation. Share your positive thoughts with others and you will bring energy and happiness to both them and yourself. Tell others when they look nice or they've done a good job. This kind of positivity can be infectious and will benefit everyone.

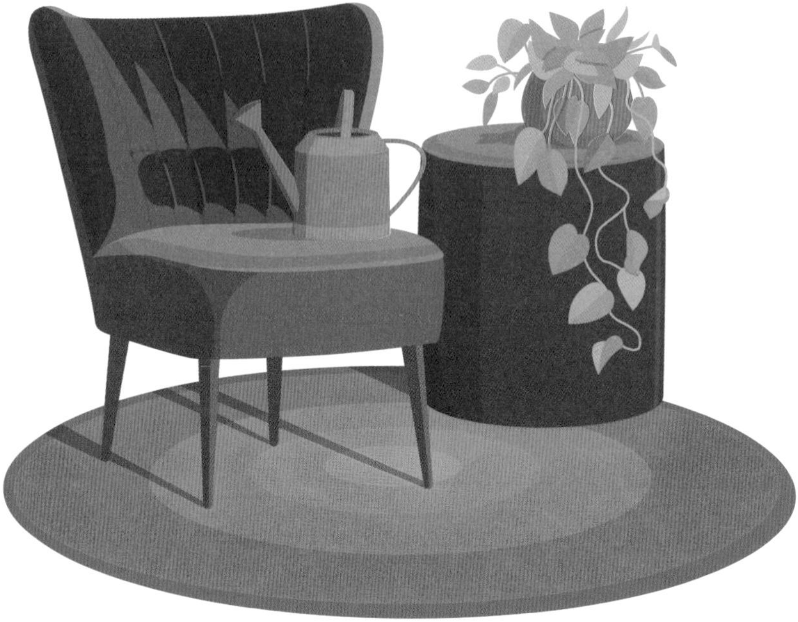

Take a break from worry

If you are concerned about something and the worry is persistent, take a break. It's hard to think clearly and solve a problem when your head is busy and cluttered with lots of different thoughts at the same time. Distract yourself for a short period of time, say for 15 or 30 minutes. Get out of the house if you can and take a walk, make yourself a hot drink or complete a chore you've been putting off for a while. Sometimes, these small distractions can help clear your mind.

Go as far as you can see; when you get there, you'll be able to see further.

Thomas Carlyle

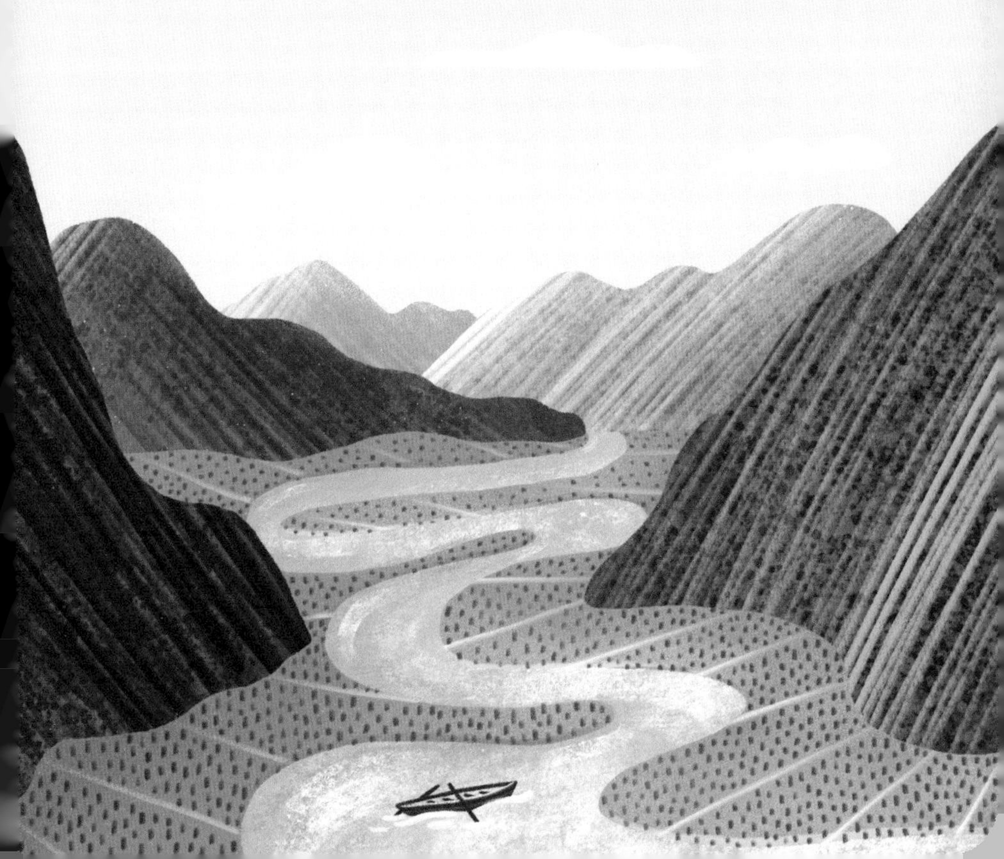

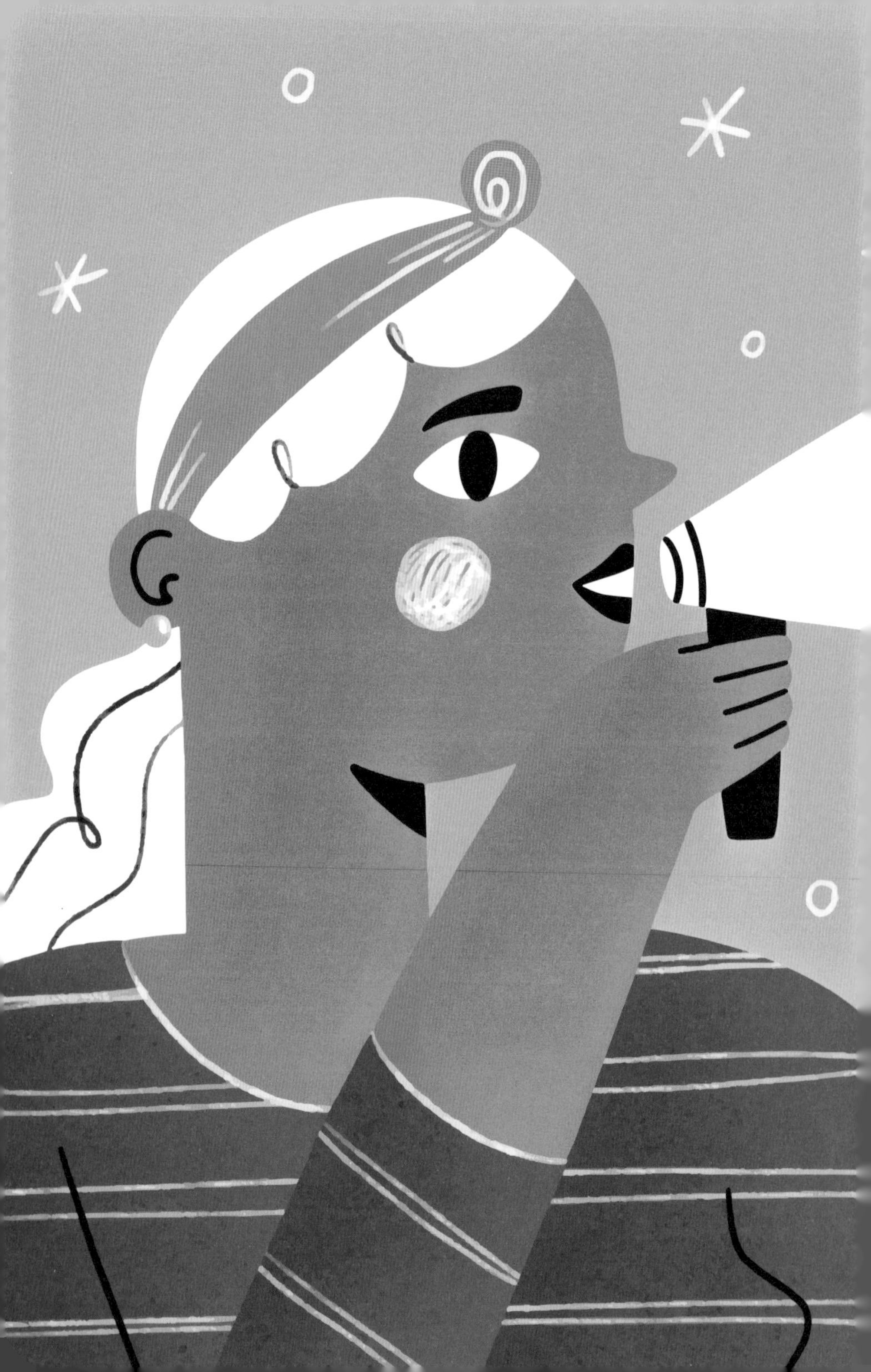

Talk it through

Understanding triggers for your anxiety can help you to manage it, and there are other ways to look at the problem too. Firstly, talking to someone you trust about how you are feeling will help. Let the person know you don't necessarily need advice (unless you feel their opinion on a situation would help) but simply want to talk about how you feel. Even if it doesn't solve your problems it will help to know that someone else understands. If you feel like you can't stop worrying, rather than trying to ignore your worries, set aside some time to focus on them so that you can seriously question whether they are justified. Write down your concerns about a situation and see if you can rate them on a scale of one to ten, in terms of how serious they really are. If they score less than a six out of ten on the worry scale, then ask whether they really deserve your time and emotional energy. If your worries are more significant, then think about what you could do to move closer to easing the pressure.

Don't
sweat
the small
stuff

Learn how to prioritize

Life is precious, and the expression "Do more of what makes you happy" is worth taking on board. Make sure you prioritize the things that are most important to you. It's easy to get distracted by trying to keep up with what's going on in the world or to find you often get swept up in a daily routine without doing what matters to you. Identify the important things in your life – be it family, health, leisure – and make time for them so that you feel that your emotional and spiritual needs are being met. This will help you to feel calmer and more fulfilled, and to enjoy a more positive mindset, which in turn will help to reduce anxiety.

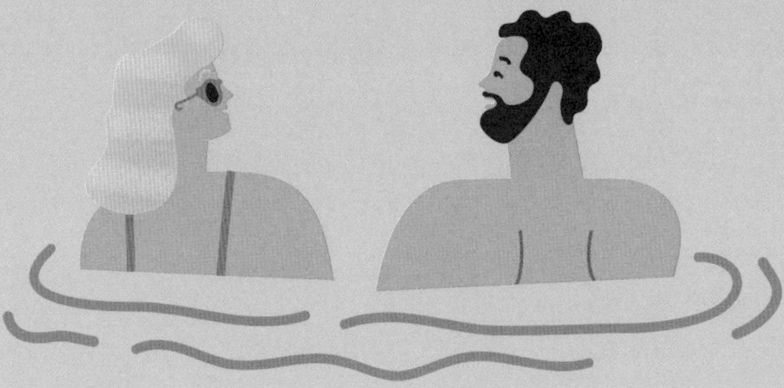

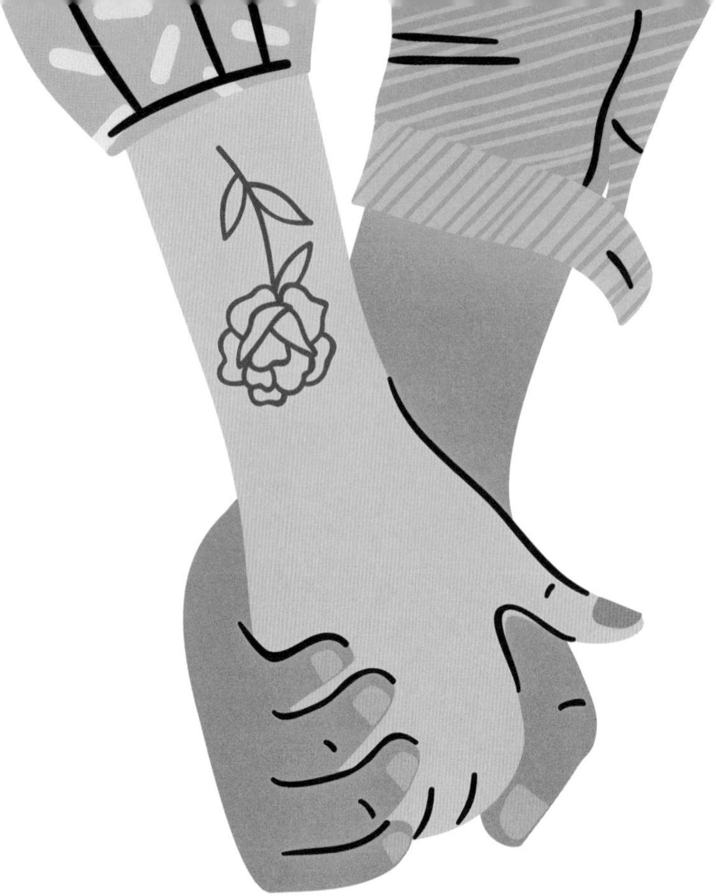

Trust in what you love,
continue to do it and it will take
you where you need to go.

Natalie Goldberg

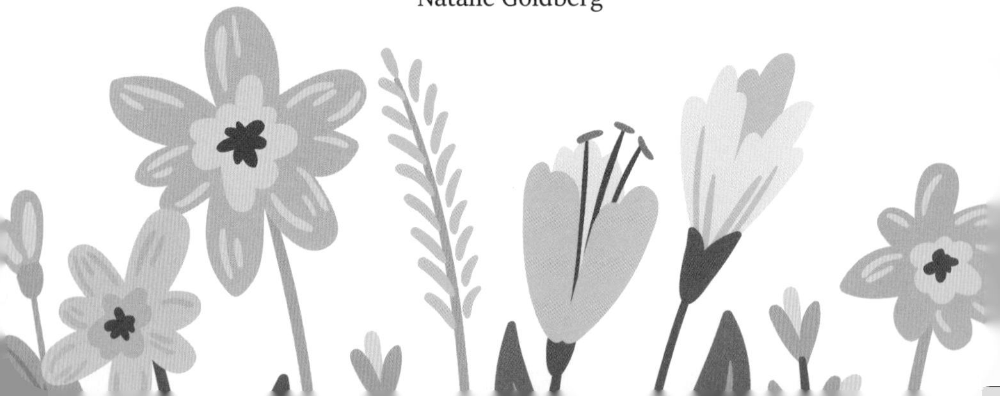

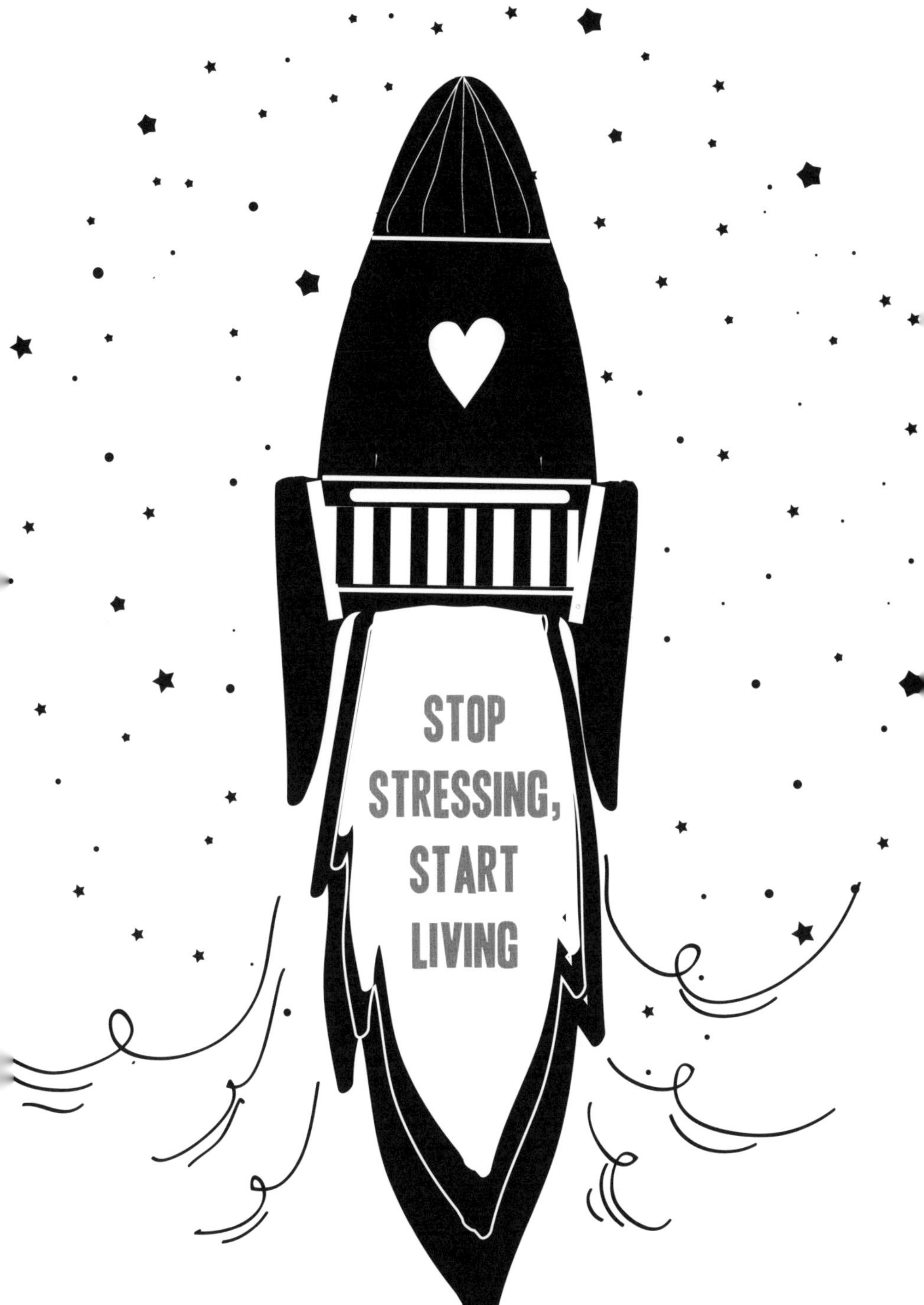
STOP
STRESSING,
START
LIVING

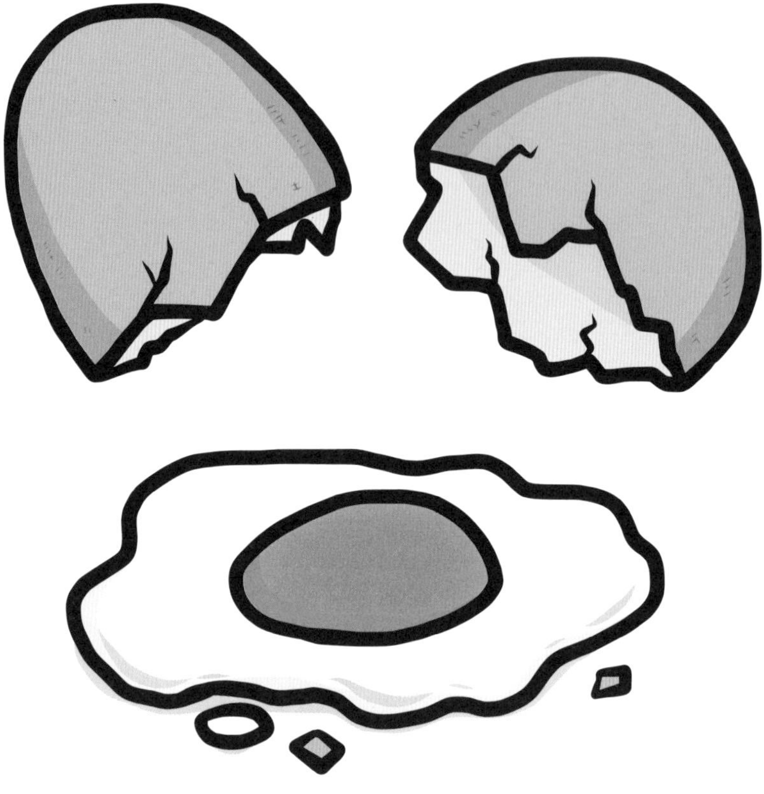

THE ONLY REAL MISTAKE WE MAKE IS THE ONE FROM WHICH WE LEARN NOTHING.

Henry Ford

Make your phone your friend

Having access to information such as emails and messages 24 hours a day can be a source of stress, especially if you've developed the habit of reading work emails just before bedtime! Make your mobile phone work for you. Instead of it being a source of possible tension, use it to improve your health and well-being: try a sleep or meditation app to help you feel calm or a fitness app to monitor your exercise and help you feel more motivated about being healthy. Make your phone work for you in a positive way rather than cluttering your mind with too many thoughts and information overload.

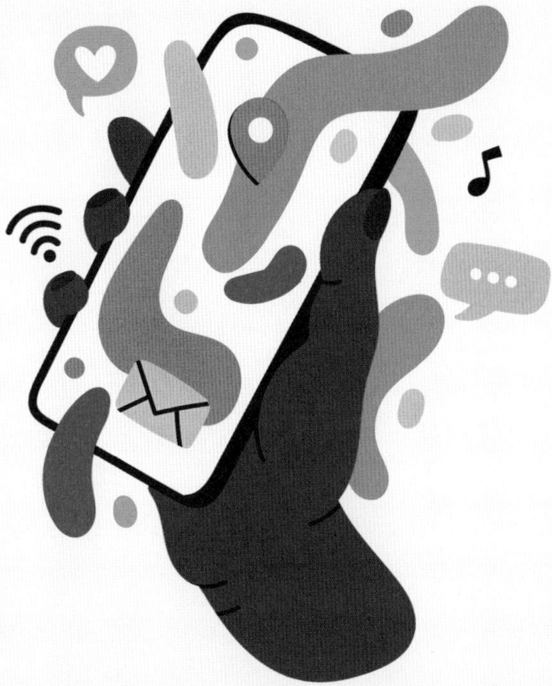

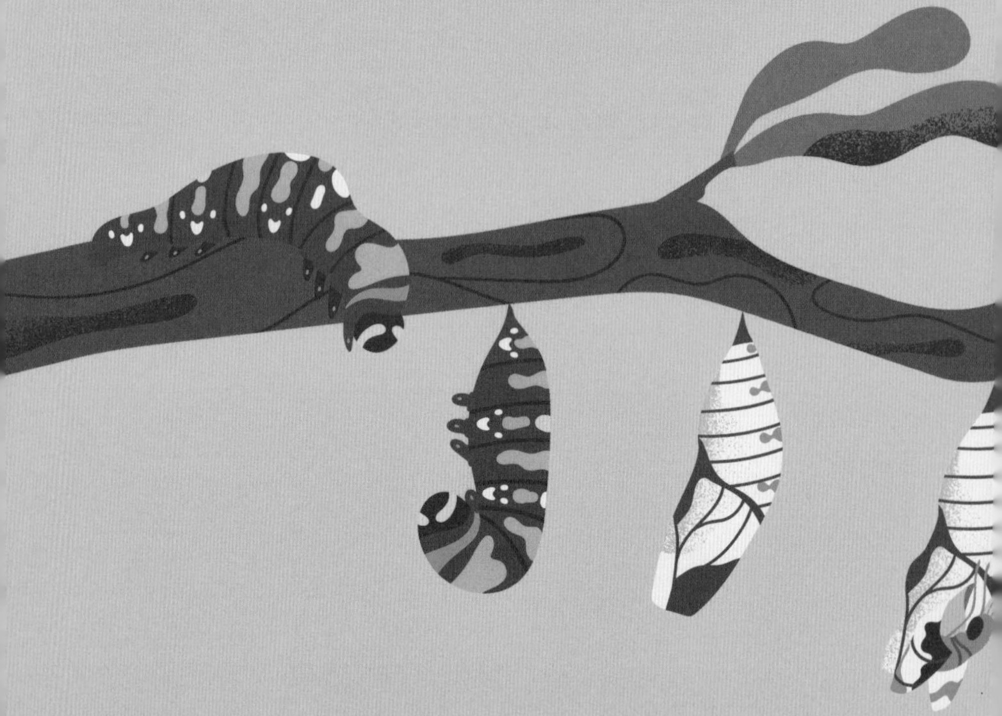

Keep evolving

If you want to feel that your life has purpose, then keep growing. Set goals and when you achieve them, set new ones. Learning new things releases dopamine, which is a chemical that transmits signals between the nerve cells of the brain and makes us feel good when we are trying something new or motivated by doing something different; it's also responsible for reward, motivation and memory, so you will feel more energized mentally. It's important to be aware that we can evolve in our mental health and well-being too.

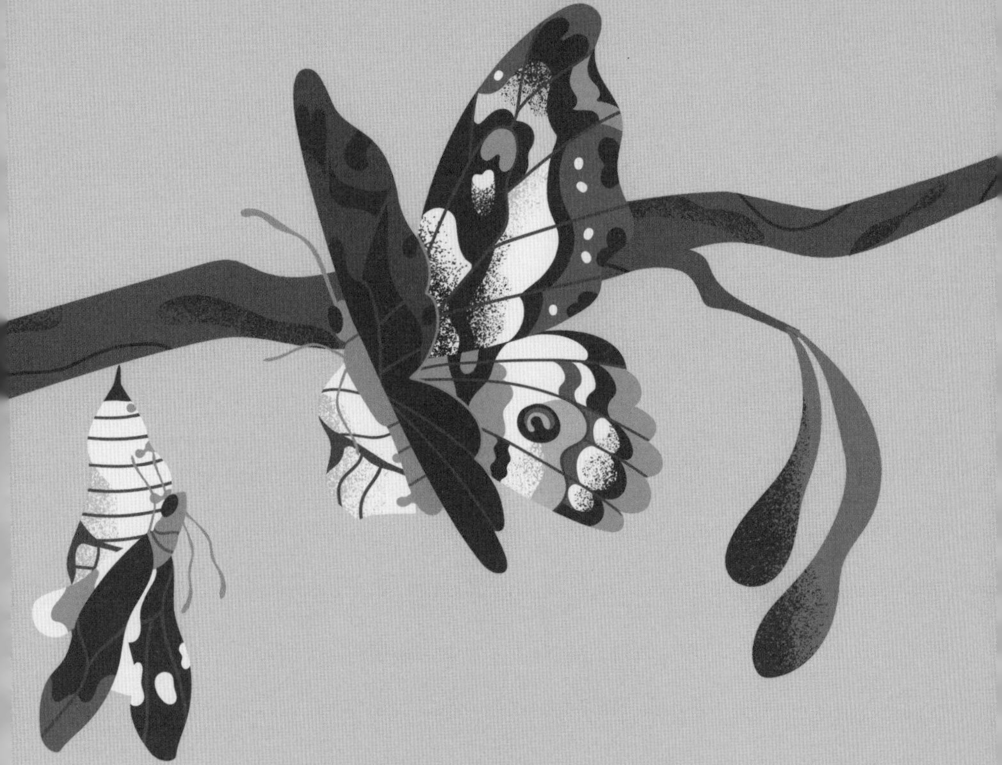

We can train ourselves to understand how our mind works and what triggers anxiety and worry. Learning to be aware of what triggers your anxious thoughts will make you better placed to manage them. Anxiety, after all, is a process and there will be many stages of the journey in controlling your mindset and managing how you deal with it. You don't have to fix everything at once though – keep learning and developing.

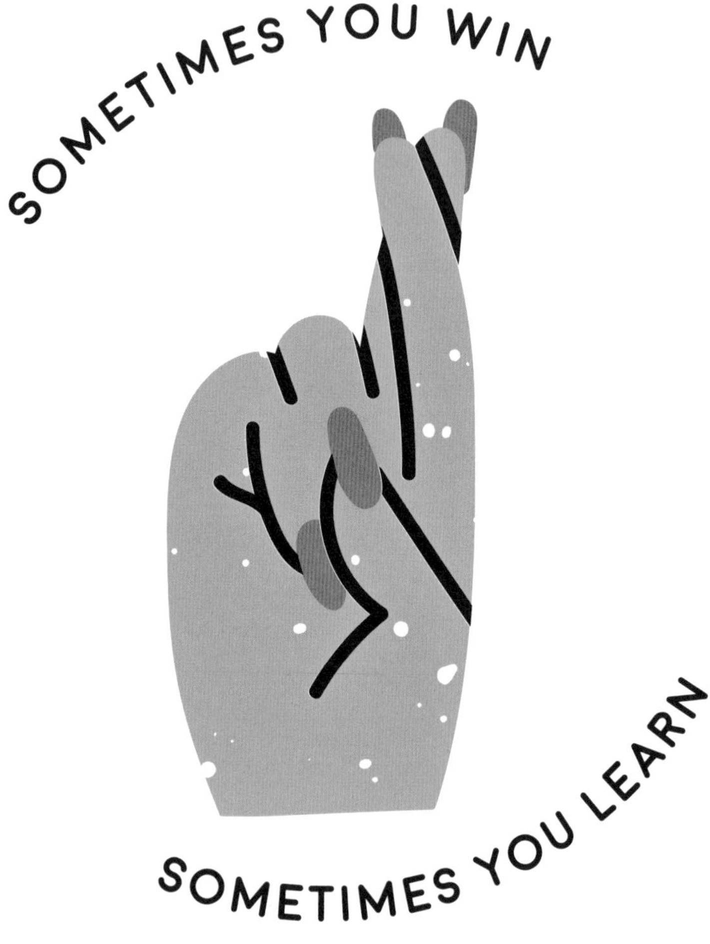
SOMETIMES YOU WIN
SOMETIMES YOU LEARN

HOWEVER DIFFICULT LIFE MAY SEEM, THERE IS ALWAYS SOMETHING YOU CAN DO AND SUCCEED AT.

Stephen Hawking

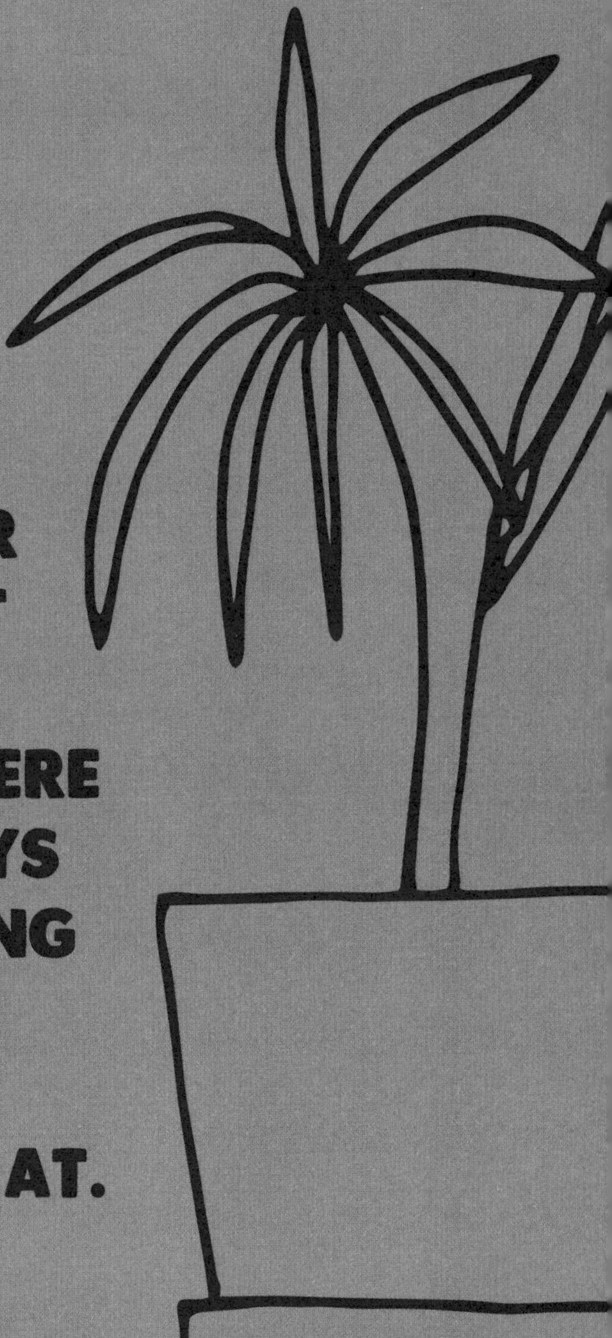

KNOWING YOURSELF IS THE BEGINNING OF ALL WISDOM

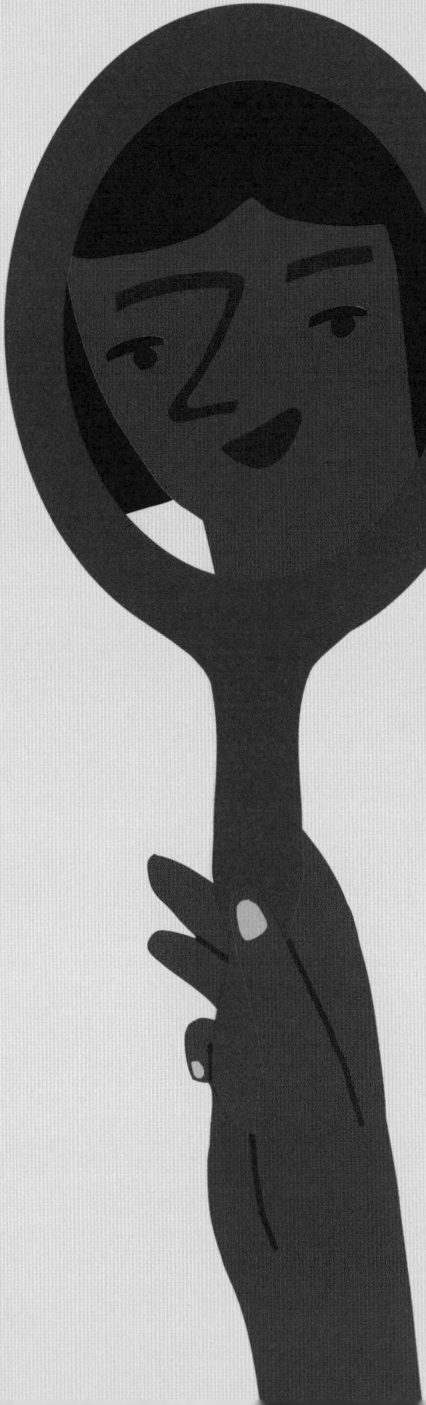

Turn anxiety into a positive

With the right frame of mind, you can turn any situation around. If, for instance, you are working long hours and this is making you feel stressed and burned out, and you know your colleagues are feeling the same, look into how you can change this. Set up initiatives in your workplace to limit the amount of overtime that staff have to carry out. Organize a lunchtime fitness class or exercise walk so that everyone has a chance to introduce some calm to their busy day. Not only will this relieve your anxiety but it will also help others.

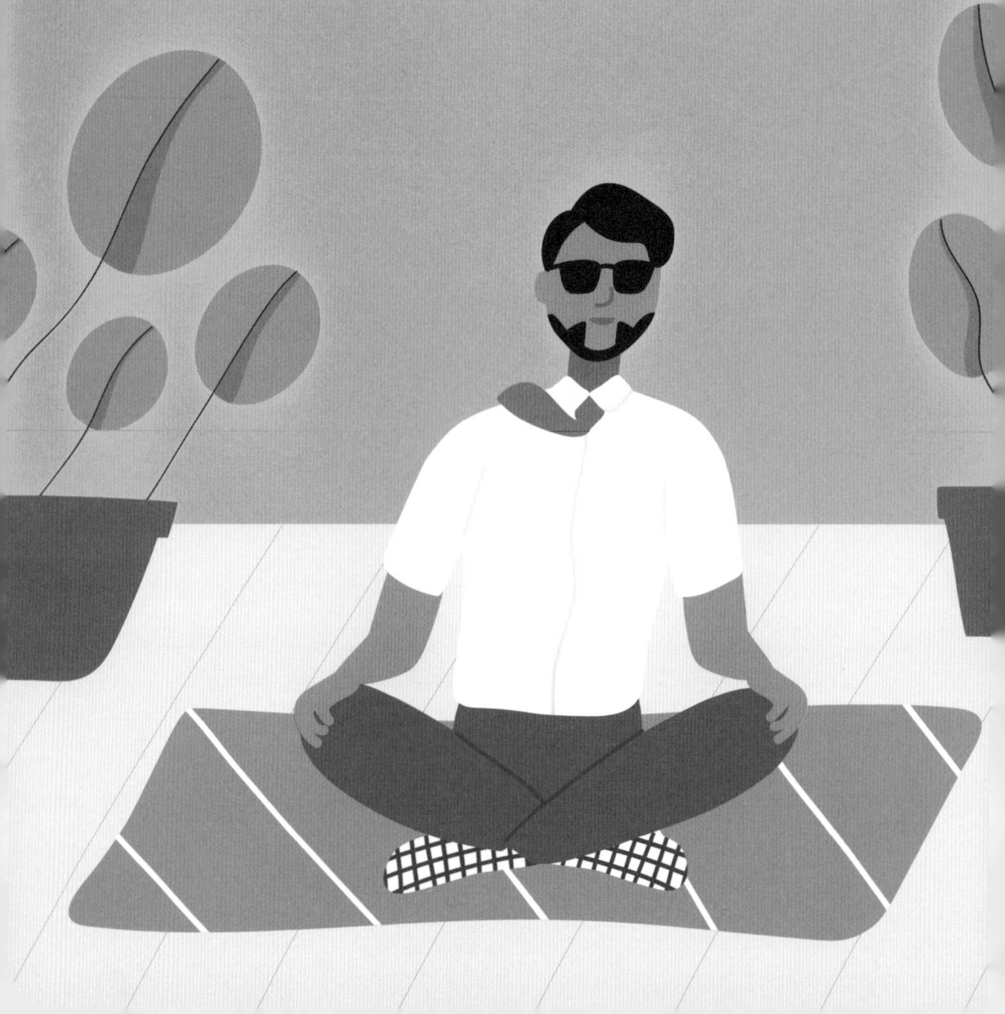

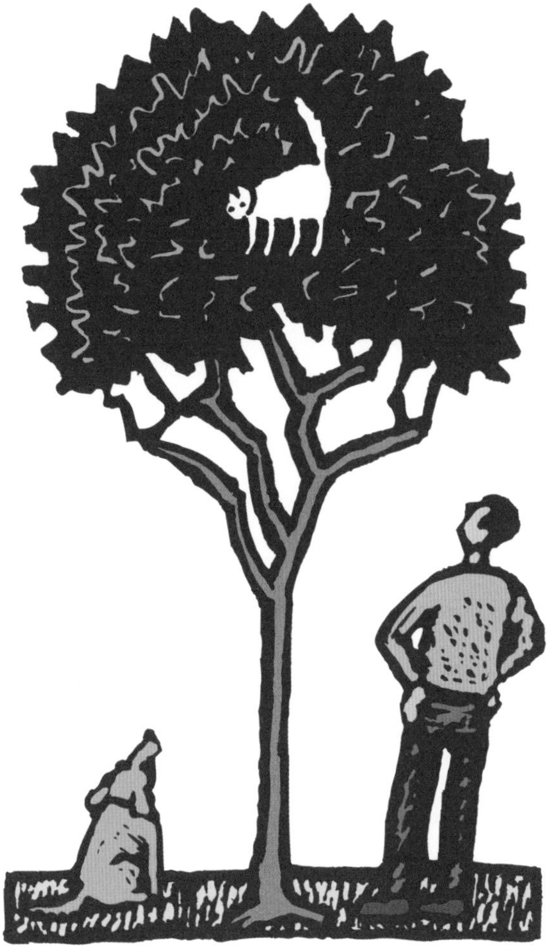

Ultimately there is no such thing as failure. There are lessons learned in different ways.

Twyla Tharp

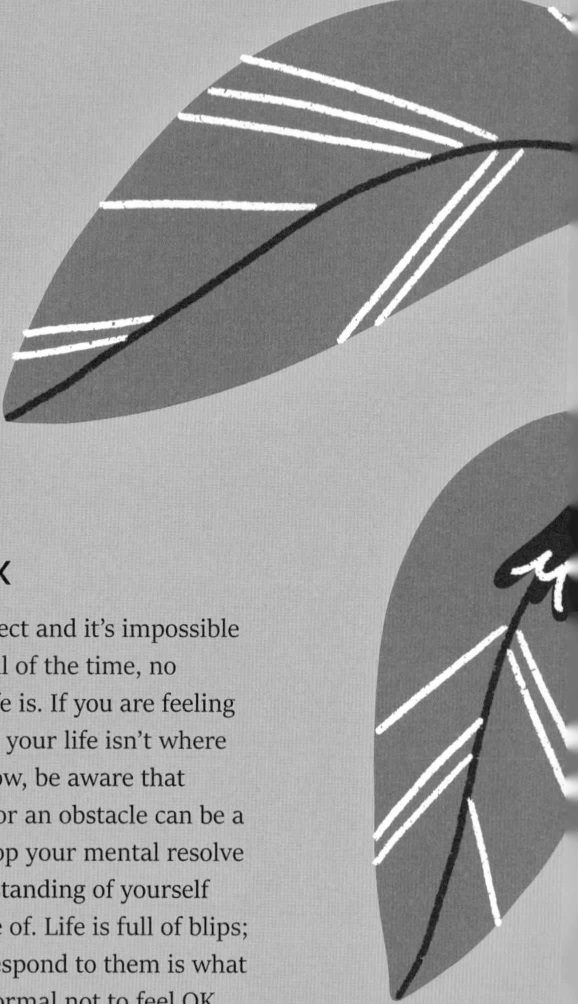

It's OK to not be OK

You don't have to be perfect and it's impossible for anyone to be happy all of the time, no matter how good their life is. If you are feeling down and frustrated that your life isn't where you want it to be right now, be aware that sometimes hitting a low or an obstacle can be a good thing – it can develop your mental resolve and improve your understanding of yourself and what you are capable of. Life is full of blips; how you deal with and respond to them is what matters. But, while it's normal not to feel OK all the time, don't ignore long-term feelings of stress, anxiety or despair, and seek help if you feel that your anxiety is spiralling out of control.

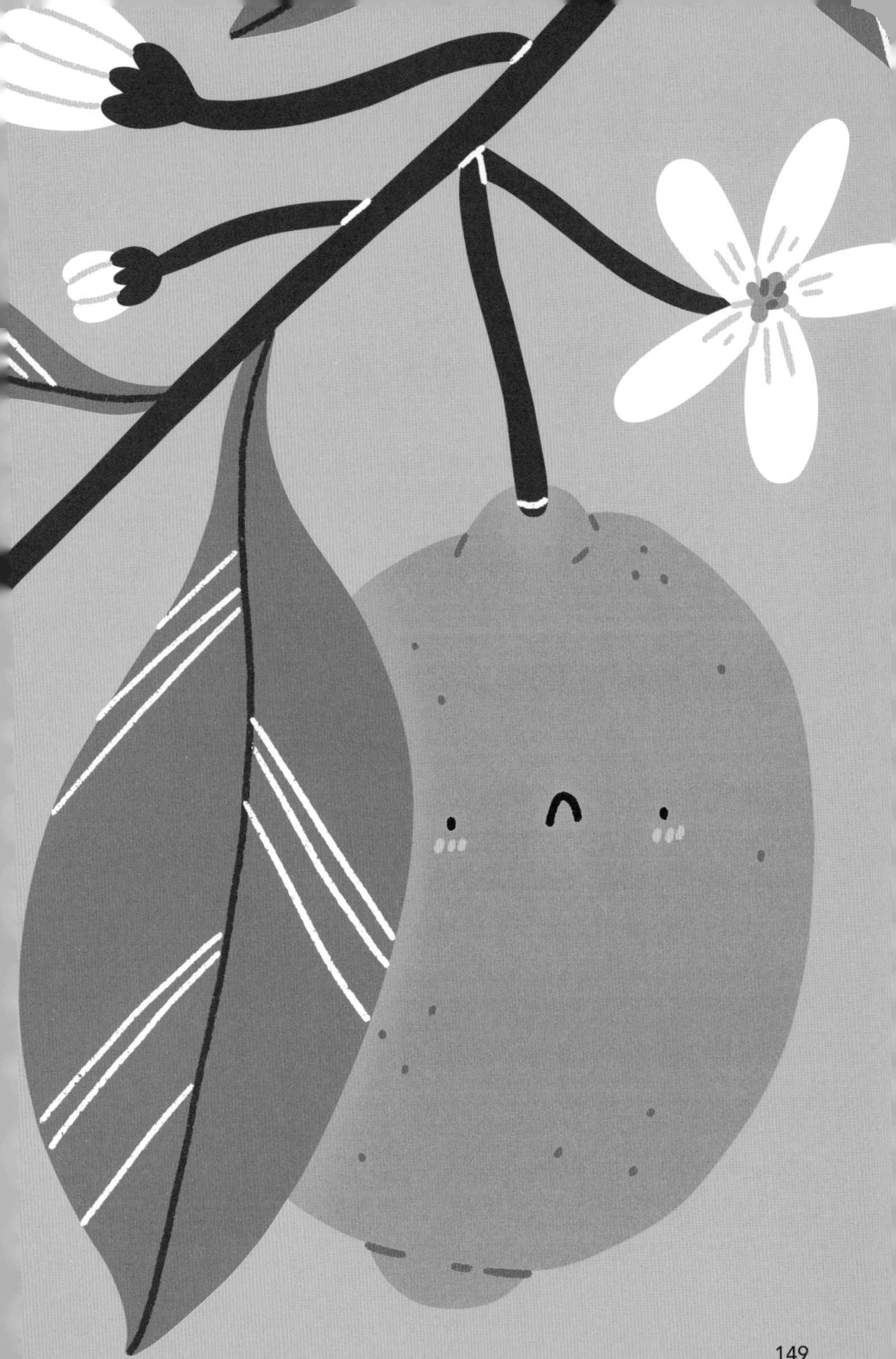

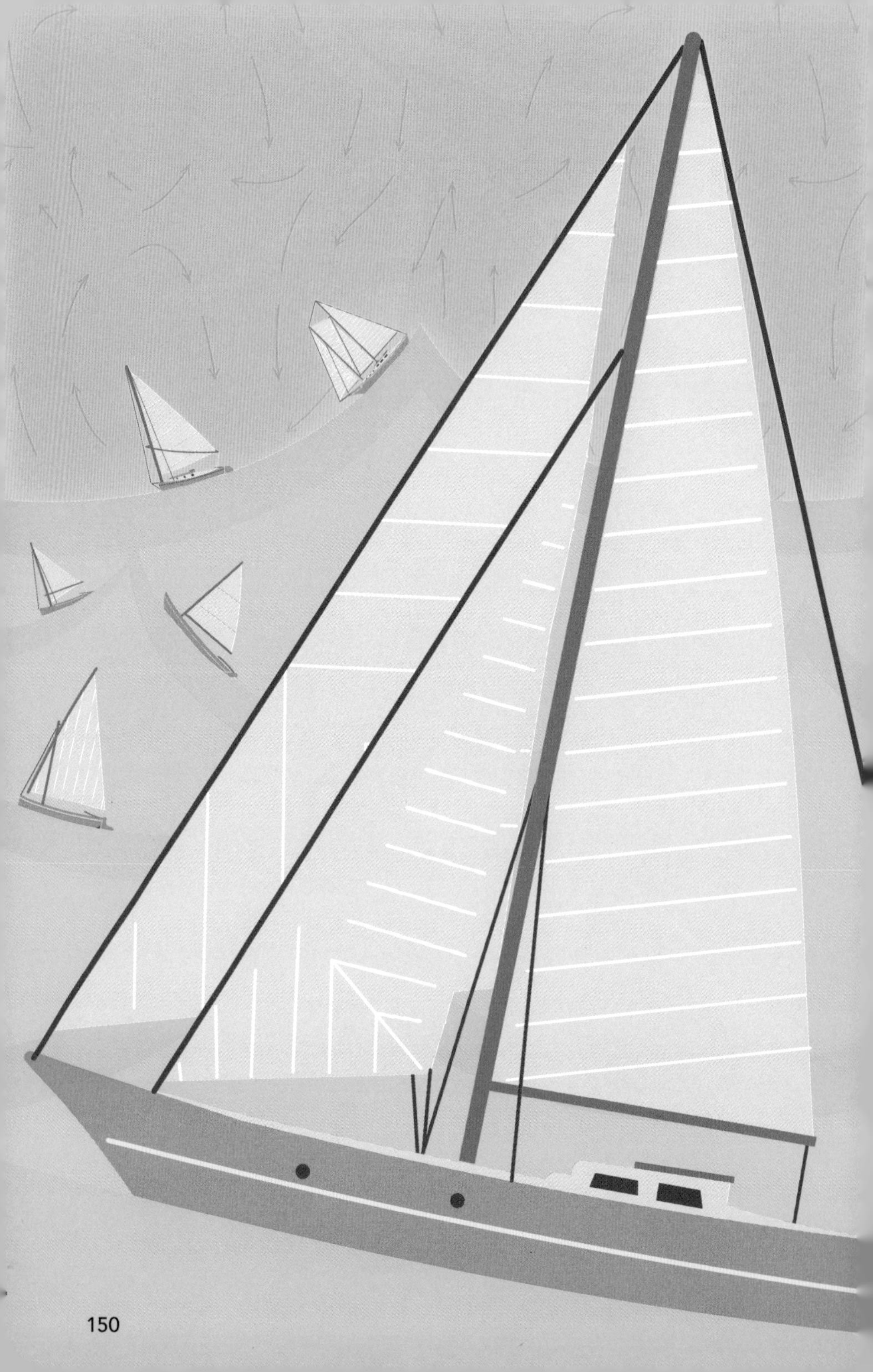

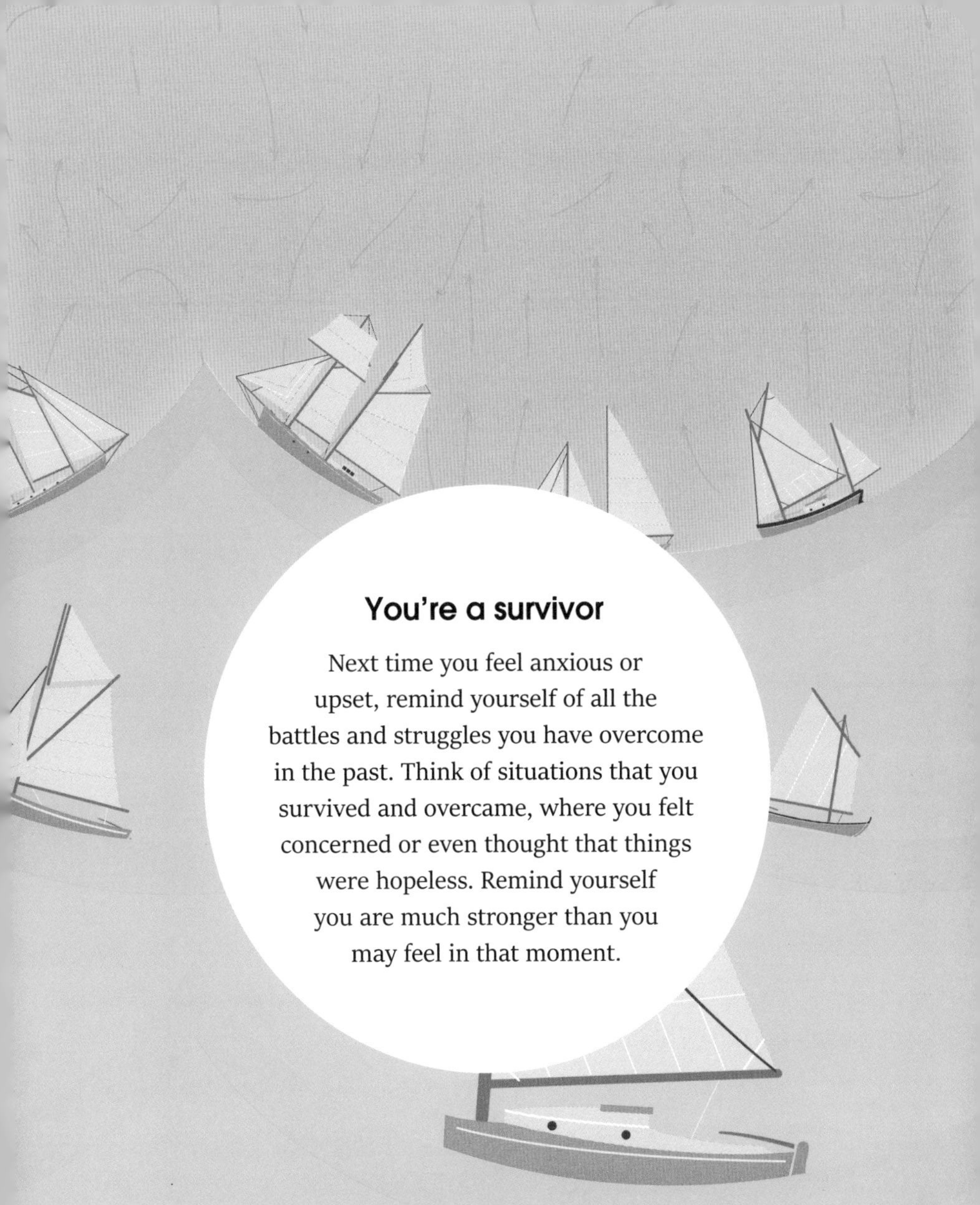

You're a survivor

Next time you feel anxious or upset, remind yourself of all the battles and struggles you have overcome in the past. Think of situations that you survived and overcame, where you felt concerned or even thought that things were hopeless. Remind yourself you are much stronger than you may feel in that moment.

Try Cognitive Behavioural Therapy

Cognitive Behavioural Therapy (CBT) is a talking therapy that focuses on your thoughts and beliefs and how they affect your behaviour. It may be useful if you have unresolved issues from your past. You work with a therapist to identify and challenge negative thinking patterns and overcome them, teaching you how to develop coping skills for dealing with situations and problems. CBT is used to treat anxiety and depression and can also be applied to treat panic disorder, phobias and bipolar disorder, to name a few. The aim is for you to apply the skills you have learned to everyday life, to encourage you to handle negative thinking.

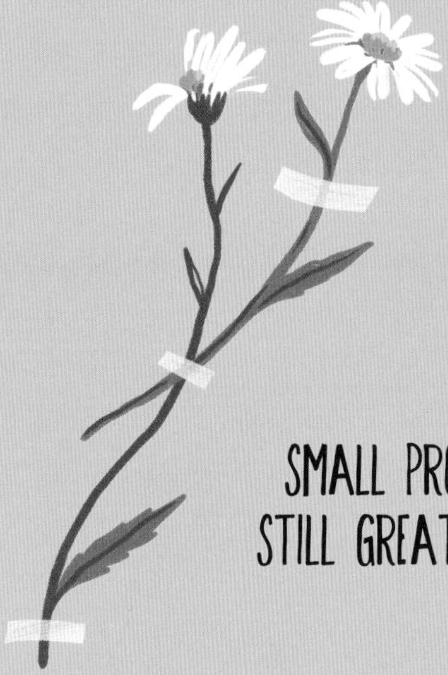

SMALL PROGRESS IS
STILL GREAT PROGRESS

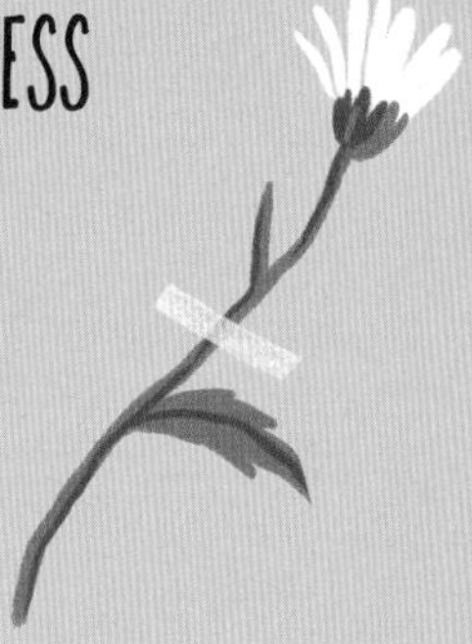

Connect with others in similar situations

If you are going through hard times, or you're simply feeling stressed or concerned, teaming up with others who are going through a similar experience or are in a similar situation to you could help you to feel calmer. For instance, carers often find comfort in talking to other carers about the challenges they face, because they know that other carers understand exactly how they feel. Talking to well-meaning friends may help, but in some cases your friends may not understand what you are experiencing. Consider joining a support group – there are many online communities for depression, anxiety and other mental health issues. Sometimes we don't need someone to solve our problems; we can gain a lot of comfort and strength from simply knowing that there are others out there who understand our challenges.

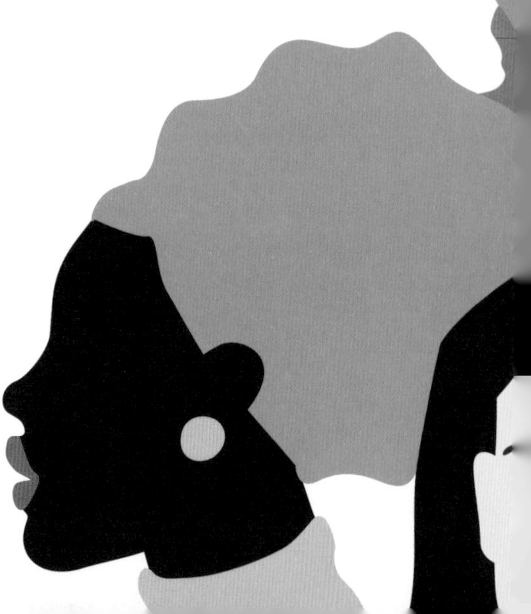

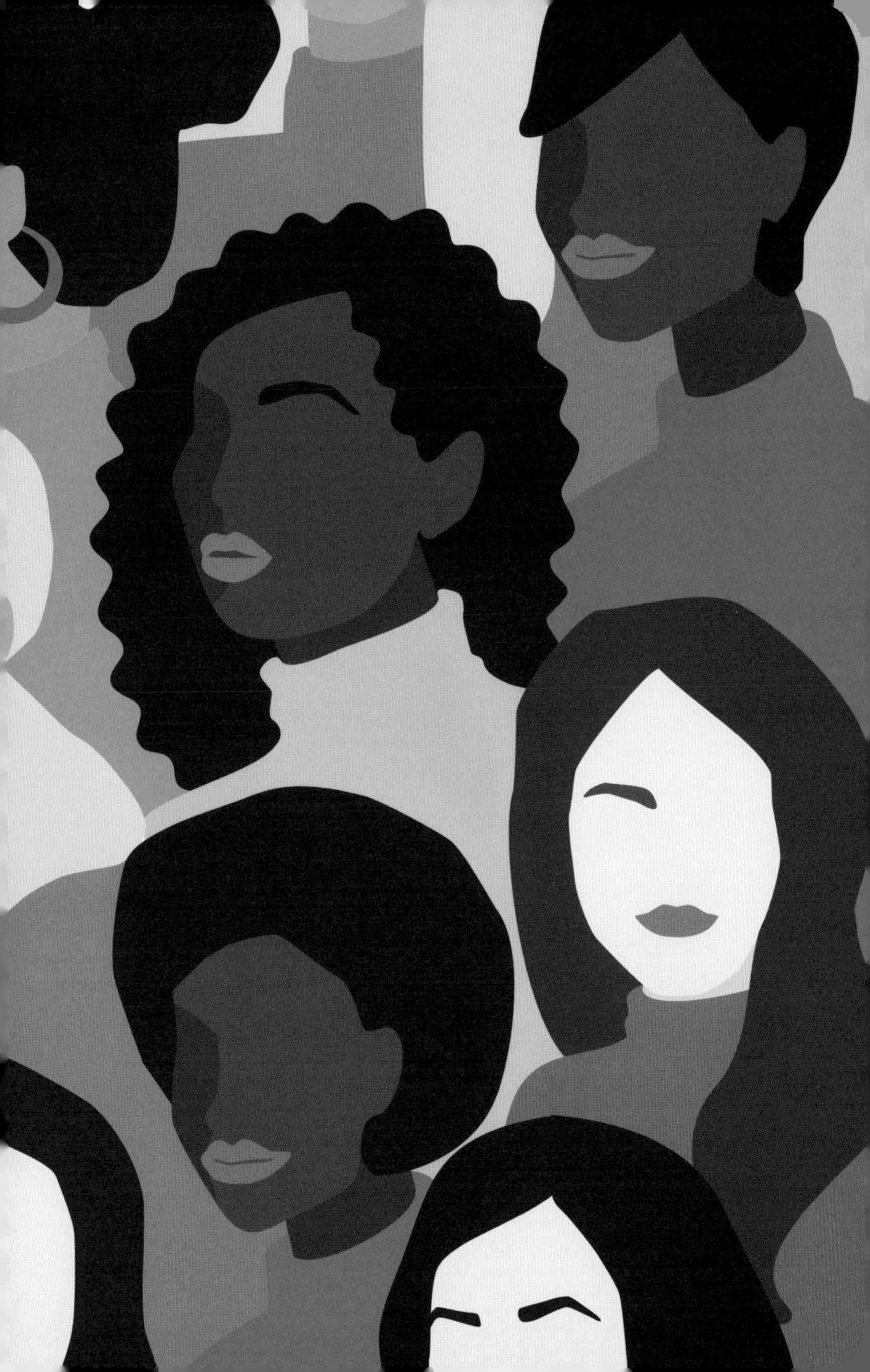

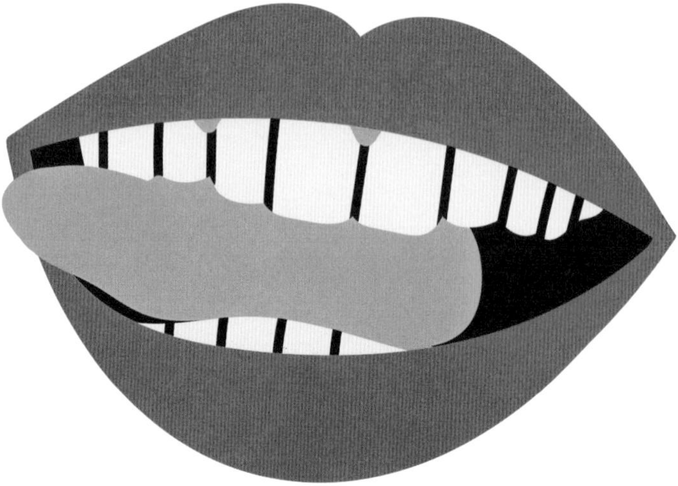

Tell yourself when to stop

If you feel your thoughts starting to spiral out of control in relation to a situation that is worrying you, and you find yourself thinking negatively, in your mind shout "Stop!" Tell yourself you are not going down that road again. It may sound simple, but it can be incredibly effective. Take some deep breaths and refocus – maybe by talking to someone else who may have a more grounded and less emotional reaction to what's going on.

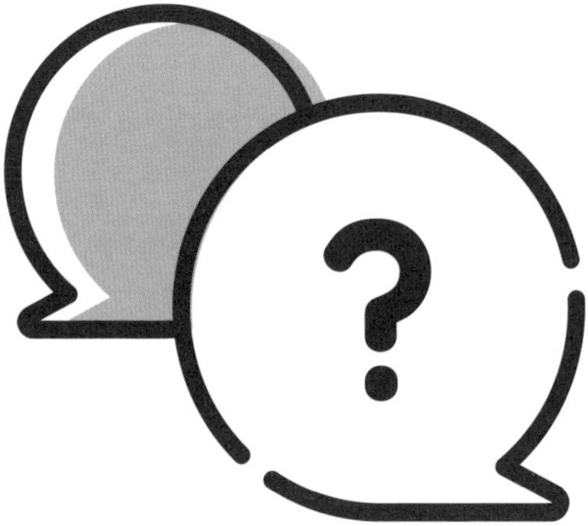

Medical Advice

If you have reached the end of this book and tried the ideas and techniques within, but still feel like you are unable to achieve a quieter mind, it may be the right time to seek professional help. Book an appointment with your GP to see what they recommend. Remember to tell them everything; there is nothing they haven't heard before. The more honest you are and the more detail you give, the more you give your GP a better chance of finding a treatment that will work for you.

Conclusion

Don't Give Up – Take Control

Congratulations on taking the first steps to improve self-awareness and take control of your mind! Hopefully this book has helped you realize that there are many ways of dealing with anxiety – from challenging negative thoughts to taking regular exercise, getting good quality sleep and minimizing digital distractions. A key point is to be aware that you can take control of stress – even if you face situations that can't be immediately resolved, you can change how you respond to them and use some of the tips and tricks in this book to calm your mind and think more clearly. While you don't have to get everything right from the get-go, and working on your mindset takes time and is an evolving process, knowing that you're taking action and doing things to combat your anxiety may, in itself, make you feel better. We all like to feel that we're in control of our lives, and taking positive action is the first step to improving your mood and sense of ownership over your life. Remember that self-improvement is an ongoing process, so long may it continue.

Image Credits

p.2 © photolinc, Violetta Smoliankina/Shutterstock.com; p.3 © Alenka Karabanova/Shutterstock.com; pp.4–5 © Wanda Pelin Canila/Shutterstock.com; pp.6–8 © abstract_art7/Shutterstock.com; p.9 © Nicetoseeya/ Shutterstock.com; pp.10–11 © Alenka Karabanova/Shutterstock.com; p.12 © Undrey/Shutterstock.com; p.14 © Alenka Karabanova/Shutterstock.com; p.15 © Alenka Karabanova/Shutterstock.com; pp.16–17 © Alenka Karabanova/Shutterstock.com; p.18 © Alenka Karabanova/Shutterstock.com; p.19 © Alenka Karabanova/ Shutterstock.com; p.21 © mhatzapa/Shutterstock.com; p.22 © Alenka Karabanova/Shutterstock.com; p.23 © Alenka Karabanova/Shutterstock.com; p.24 © GoodStudio/Shutterstock.com; p.27 © GoodStudio/ Shutterstock.com; p.28 © Alenka Karabanova/Shutterstock.com; pp.30–31 © Violetta Smoliankina/ Shutterstock.com; p.32 © Novak Viataha/Shutterstock.com; p.33 © Julia August/Shutterstock.com; p.34 © Bibadash/Shutterstock.com; p.35 © Katflare/Shutterstock.com; pp.36–37 © Ksenia Loginovskikh/ Shutterstock.com; p.38 © Piyapong89/Shutterstock.com; p.39 © Piyapong89/Shutterstock.com; pp.40–41 © Violetta Smoliankina/Shutterstock.com; p.42 © Spirit Boom Cat/Shutterstock.com; p.43 © Alenka Karabanova/Shutterstock.com; pp.44–45 © Spirit Boom Cat/Shutterstock.com; p.47 © Nicetoseeya/ Shutterstock.com; p.48 © norph/Shutterstock.com; p.49 © GoodStudio/Shutterstock.com; p.50 © Spirit Boom Cat/Shutterstock.com; pp.52–53 © Bibadash/Shutterstock.com; p.54 © Alenka Karabanova/ Shutterstock.com; p.55 © Bibadash/Shutterstock.com; p.56 © cosmaa/Shutterstock.com; pp.58–59 © Tithi Luadthong/Shutterstock.com; p.60 © GoodStudio/Shutterstock.com; p.61 © liskus/Shutterstock.com; pp.64–65 © Viktoria Kurpas/Shutterstock.com; p.66 © PACPUMI/Shutterstock.com; p.67 © Lera Efremova/ Shutterstock.com; p.68 © Nata9/Shutterstock.com; p.69 © Piyapong89/Shutterstock.com; p.70 © Bibadash/ Shutterstock.com; p.71 © Olha Turchenko/Shutterstock.com; p.72 © Piyapong89/Shutterstock.com; p.73 © Ohn Mar/Shutterstock.com; p.74 © owatta/Shutterstock.com; p.76 © PACPUMI/Shutterstock.com; p.79 © Bibadash/Shutterstock.com; p.80 © Arkadivna/Shutterstock.com; p.81 © GoodStudio/Shutterstock. com; p.83 © Nadia Grapes/Shutterstock.com; p.85 © CreativeUniverse/Shutterstock.com; p.86 © Violetta Smoliankina/Shutterstock.com; p.87 © sinoptic/Shutterstock.com; p.88 © owatta/Shutterstock.com; p.89 © Alenka Karabanova/Shutterstock.com; p.91 © Bibadash/Shutterstock.com; pp.92–93 © Marish/Shutterstock. com; p.95 © cosmaa/Shutterstock.com; p.97 © owatta/Shutterstock.com; p.98 © Kolesnikov Vladimir/ Shutterstock.com; p.99 © GoodStudio/Shutterstock.com; p.101 © Nicetoseeya/Shutterstock.com; p.102 © owatta/Shutterstock.com; p.103 © Alenka Karabanova/Shutterstock.com; p.104 © Double Brain/Shutterstock. com; p.105 © Ksusha Dusmikeeva/Shutterstock.com; pp.106–107 © Alenka Karabanova/Shutterstock.com; pp.108–109 © GoodStudio/Shutterstock.com; p.110 © Novak Viataha/Shutterstock.com; p.111 © owatta/ Shutterstock.com; p.112 © Katrine Glazkova/Shutterstock.com; p.113 © Ksusha Dusmikeeva/Shutterstock. com; p.115 © Nicetoseeya/Shutterstock.com; p.116 © Ksusha Dusmikeeva/Shutterstock.com; p.117 © Nicetoseeya/Shutterstock.com; p.118 © Novak Viataha/Shutterstock.com; p.119 © Ksusha Dusmikeeva/ Shutterstock.com; p.120 © owatta/Shutterstock.com; p.121 © cosmaa/Shutterstock.com; p.122 © PACPUMI/ Shutterstock.com; p.123 © Novak Viataha/Shutterstock.com; p.124–125 © Novak Viataha/Shutterstock.com; p.126–127 © Zenzen/Shutterstock.com; p.128 © owatta/Shutterstock.com; p.129 © owatta/Shutterstock.com; p.130 © Dotidrop/Shutterstock.com; p.131 © Ksusha Dusmikeeva/Shutterstock.com; pp.132–133© Ksusha Dusmikeeva/Shutterstock.com; p.135© Nicetoseeya/Shutterstock.com; p.136 © Nadia Grapes/Shutterstock. com; p.137 © Hanna Kh/Shutterstock.com; p.138 © owatta/Shutterstock.com; p.139 © Bibadash/ Shutterstock.com; pp.140–141 © GoodStudio/Shutterstock.com; p.142 © Bibadash/Shutterstock.com; p.143 © Elena Novi/Shutterstock.com; p.145 © Nicetoseeya/Shutterstock.com; p.146 © GoodStudio/Shutterstock.com; p.147 © Ron and Joe/Shutterstock.com; pp.148–149 © Ksusha Dusmikeeva/Shutterstock.com; pp.150–151 © Spirit Boom Cat/Shutterstock.com; p.152 © Nicetoseeya/Shutterstock.com; p.153 © Alenka Karabanova/ Shutterstock.com; pp.154–155 © Nadia Grapes/Shutterstock.com; p.156 © Bibadash/Shutterstock.com; p.157 © Introwiz1/Shutterstock.com; p.158 © Bibadash/Shutterstock.com; p.160 © ChalidMGM/Shutterstock.com